CAMBRIDGE LIBRARY COLLECTION

Books of enduring scholarly value

History

The books reissued in this series include accounts of historical events and movements by eye-witnesses and contemporaries, as well as landmark studies that assembled significant source materials or developed new historiographical methods. The series includes work in social, political and military history on a wide range of periods and regions, giving modern scholars ready access to influential publications of the past.

Chapters on Mental Physiology

Sir Henry Holland (1788–1873), physician and travel writer, was one of the best known and sought-after doctors in nineteenth-century Britain. He was medical attendant to Queen Caroline, the wife of George IV, and was appointed physician-extraordinary to Queen Victoria on her accession in 1837. Holland also counted six British prime ministers among his patients. He received honorary degrees from Oxford and Harvard, and served as president of the Royal Society three times. First published in 1852, Holland's book on mental physiology explores the medical links between mind and body, including the ways in which sleep, insanity, memory, age, instincts, and habits affect the human body and nervous system. Parts of this work also appeared in Holland's earlier publication, *Medical Notes and Reflections* (1839). While many of the theories on which he writes (such as phrenology) have since been discredited, Holland's book remains an intriguing insight into Victorian medical science.

Cambridge University Press has long been a pioneer in the reissuing of out-of-print titles from its own backlist, producing digital reprints of books that are still sought after by scholars and students but could not be reprinted economically using traditional technology. The Cambridge Library Collection extends this activity to a wider range of books which are still of importance to researchers and professionals, either for the source material they contain, or as landmarks in the history of their academic discipline.

Drawing from the world-renowned collections in the Cambridge University Library, and guided by the advice of experts in each subject area, Cambridge University Press is using state-of-the-art scanning machines in its own Printing House to capture the content of each book selected for inclusion. The files are processed to give a consistently clear, crisp image, and the books finished to the high quality standard for which the Press is recognised around the world. The latest print-on-demand technology ensures that the books will remain available indefinitely, and that orders for single or multiple copies can quickly be supplied.

The Cambridge Library Collection will bring back to life books of enduring scholarly value (including out-of-copyright works originally issued by other publishers) across a wide range of disciplines in the humanities and social sciences and in science and technology.

Chapters on
Mental Physiology

Henry Holland

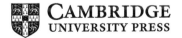

CAMBRIDGE
UNIVERSITY PRESS

CAMBRIDGE UNIVERSITY PRESS

Cambridge, New York, Melbourne, Madrid, Cape Town,
Singapore, São Paolo, Delhi, Tokyo, Mexico City

Published in the United States of America by Cambridge University Press, New York

www.cambridge.org
Information on this title: www.cambridge.org/9781108037938

© in this compilation Cambridge University Press 2011

This edition first published 1852
This digitally printed version 2011

ISBN 978-1-108-03793-8 Paperback

CHAPTERS

ON

MENTAL PHYSIOLOGY.

London :
Spottiswoodes and Shaw,
New-street-Square.

CHAPTERS

ON

MENTAL PHYSIOLOGY.

BY

HENRY HOLLAND, M.D. F.R.S. &c. &c.,

FELLOW OF THE ROYAL COLLEGE OF PHYSICIANS,
PHYSICIAN EXTRAORDINARY TO THE QUEEN,
AND PHYSICIAN IN ORDINARY TO H.R.H. PRINCE ALBERT.

FOUNDED CHIEFLY ON

CHAPTERS CONTAINED IN " MEDICAL NOTES AND REFLECTIONS,"

BY THE SAME AUTHOR.

Ὅσα γὰρ τὴν τῶν ὀμμάτων ὄψιν ἐκφεύγει, ταῦτα τῇ τῆς γνώμης ὄψει
κεκράτηται.—HIPPOCRATES.

LONDON:

LONGMAN, BROWN, GREEN, AND LONGMANS.

1852.

PREFACE.

SOME explanation is necessary of the title and plan of this volume, that the reader may rightly apprehend not only the objects proposed, but also the method adopted to fulfil them.

The title will be understood as expressing that particular part of Human Physiology, which comprises the reciprocal actions and relations of mental and bodily phenomena, as they make up the totality of life. I need not dwell on the great interest of this subject. It is attested, as every part of this volume will show, not solely by the natural and healthy conditions of existence, but even more remarkably by those of disorder and disease. Scarcely can we name a morbid affection of body in which some feeling or function of mind is not concurrently engaged — directly or indirectly — as cause or as effect. No physician can rightly fulfil his duties without an adequate knowledge of, and constant regard to, these important relations.

I have adopted the title of Chapters on Physiology; partly to avoid the profession of a complete treatise, which this is not; — partly to indicate that most of these topics, and even their titles, are taken from another work, the first edition of which was published thirteen years ago. Those who may have read my " Medical Notes and Reflections," will perhaps recollect such Chapters, as occurring in different parts of a volume chiefly devoted to subjects more strictly medical in character. Thus interposed, however, among the latter, they were deficient in the sequence and connexion naturally belonging to the topics they treat of; and which may be considered almost indispensable to a thorough understanding of the subject.

This deficiency I have sought to supply in the present volume by bringing these several Chapters into one series; and by adding others which have appeared necessary to the completion of the plan proposed.* While preserving the titles of those de-

---

* These new chapters were originally intended for a second volume of my former work; but I have thought it better to place them here, as well from their close connexion with the other subjects treated of, as also from a doubt I entertain as to the publication of a second volume in the same form as the first. Though happily there are many reasons justifying the hope that this work has been useful to the profession, yet I am led to consider it as a fault in the original plan, that the subjects are too numerous, and too little connected in series, for that ready reference, which it is important both for the author and his readers to obtain.

A few words more I may be permitted to add regarding this former work. In selecting the subjects for it, I chose those especially

rived from my former work, and following the same general train of reasoning to the same conclusions in each, I must mention that they have been almost wholly rewritten, and very materially enlarged; such alterations and additions being made necessary, partly for the connexion of the subjects thus brought into closer association; principally from the recent accessions of knowledge on numerous points having express relation to them. Even since the last edition of my "Medical Notes," the rapid progress of Physiology — ever blending itself more closely with the general laws and inductions of physical science — has converted into certainty many things which could then be offered only as surmises, unsupported by any direct proof.

which, as involving general relations, not perhaps sufficiently regarded, seemed best adapted to suggest new views as to the causes, character, and treatment of disease. In the discussion of the subjects so chosen, the plan of the volume limited me to certain general principles and outlines of inquiry. But I still entertain the hope that some of these topics may be more fully examined by other writers; and under this view I venture to suggest a few of the Chapters, which seem especially to admit of such larger discussion. I would name the following: "On Hereditary Diseases;" "On Morbid Actions of Intermittent Kind;" "On the Connexion of certain Diseases;" "On Diseases commonly occurring but once in Life;" "On the Influence of Weather in relation to Disease;" "On disturbed Balance of Circulation and Metastasis of Disease." And to these I would willingly add (though I have myself applied the hypothesis only to the Indian Cholera) the general question regarding the *Influence of Organic Matter in the atmosphere as a cause of disease* — a subject which I feel assured will hereafter gain greatly in importance, and illustrate many points in pathology, hitherto unexplained or obscure.

Much of course will be found in this volume which is familiar to those who have studied the subject, especially of late years. But, if I do not deceive myself, there are still certain facts not heretofore duly recognised or defined, and certain relations of phenomena requiring fuller illustration than they have yet received. These I have sought to embody in the ensuing Chapters, in the order which seems best calculated to give connexion and unity to the whole. To arrange under new combinations what is already known to us, is often in itself a source of fresh knowledge, or a valuable means of correcting previous error. Various instances to this effect will, I trust, occur to the reader in his progress through the volume. I may add, that in the discussion of the subjects, though obliged to adopt certain divisions for the sake of clearness, I have kept in constant view that great law of continuity, which equally governs all mental and material phenomena. No conclusions are more secure, or more profitable, than those drawn from a careful notice of continuous relations; and of those gradations of change, which bring extreme cases within common laws, and reconcile anomalies with facts familiar to experience. To this I would advert, as a principle I have largely applied in every part of the volume.

The topics treated of are such in their nature as

perpetually to bring us to the very confines of metaphysical speculation. Except in the case of one great question, which could not be put aside, I have carefully avoided passing over this boundary. Convinced of the general truth of the maxim, that "it is safer and easier to proceed from ignorance to knowledge than from error," I have endeavoured throughout to separate what is known from that which is unknown — what is capable of being reached by the human understanding from that which is presumably unattainable by it. The close adherence to this principle will probably expose me to the charge of having surrounded the subject with unresolved doubts and difficulties. But I think it far better to incur this imputation, than to assume a knowledge not yet possessed, or to cover the deficiencies of reason by any mere artifices of language.

In different parts of this volume I have had occasion to advert to those Mesmeric phenomena and doctrines, and the topics collateral to them, which have drawn so largely upon public attention of late years. Having the interests of truth solely in view, it has seemed to me that such reference might most legitimately, as well as most usefully, be made, through the relation of the phenomena in question to those other parts of physiology, which I believe to explain their real nature, and the con-

CONTENTS.

xii CONTENTS.

CHAP. VIII.

CHAP. IX.

CHAP. X.

CHAP. XI.

ERRATA.

Page 44. l. 6., for " decide " read " divide."
91. l. 2. from bottom, for " immediate " read " intermediate."
129. l. 21., dele " sensorial."

CHAPTERS

ON

MENTAL PHYSIOLOGY.

CHAPTER I.

ON MEDICAL EVIDENCE.

THERE can be few better tests of a sound understanding, than the right estimation of medical evidence; so various are the complexities it presents, so numerous the sources of error. The subjects of observation are those in which Matter and Mind are concurrently concerned; — Matter under the complex and subtle organization, whence vitality and all its functions are derived; Mind in its equally mysterious relations to the organs thus formed; — both subject to numerous agencies from without, both undergoing very various changes from disease within. Individualities of each have their influence in creating difficulties, and these amongst the most arduous which beset the path of the physician.* Few cases occur strictly alike, even when the source of disorder is manifestly the same. Primary

---

* Idiosyncrasy, as arising in most cases from inappreciable causes, is the most absolute and inevitable difficulty in medical evidence; since no accumulation of instances, such as might suffice for the removal of all other doubts, can secure us wholly against this source of error.

B

causes of disease are often wholly obscured by those of
secondary kind.   Organs remote from each other by place
and function are simultaneously disturbed.   Translations
of morbid action take place from one part to another.
Nervous affections and sympathies often assume every
character of real disease.   While remedial agents are
rendered uncertain in effect by the various forms of each
disorder, by the idiosyncracies of the patient, by the difficulty of securing their equal application or transmission
into the system, and finally by the unequal quality of the
remedies themselves.

These difficulties, the solution of which gives medicine
its highest character as a science, can be adequately conceived by the medical man alone.   Neither those accustomed to legal evidence only, nor such as have pursued
physical science in its more simple material forms, can
rightly apprehend the vast difference made by the in-
troduction of the principle of life; or, yet more, of the
states and phenomena of mind, in connexion with bodily
organization.   We have here a new world of relations,
occult and complex in their nature, to be reasoned upon
and resolved; with a principle of change, moreover, ever
operating among them, which renders all conclusions liable
to a new source of error.   It is the want of this right
understanding of medical evidence, which makes the mass
of mankind so prone to be deceived by imposture of every
kind; whether it be the idle fashion as to particular
remedies; or the worse, because wider, deception of some
system, professing to have attained at once, what the
most learned and acute observers have laboured after for
ages in vain.

It must be admitted, indeed, that this matter of medical testimony is too lightly weighed by physicians themselves. Else whence the frequent description of effects and cures by agents put only once or twice upon trial; and the ready or eager belief given by those, who on other subjects, and even on the closely related questions of physiology, would instantly feel the insufficient nature of the proof.* Conclusions requiring for their authority a long average of cases, carefully selected, and freed from the many chances of error or ambiguity, are often promulgated and received upon grounds barely sufficient to warrant a repetition of the trials which first suggested them. No science, un happily, has abounded more in false statements and partial inferences; each usurping a place for the time in popular esteem; and each sanctioned by credulity, even where most dangerous in application to practice. During the last twenty years, omitting all lesser instances, I have known the rise and decline of five or six fashions in medical doctrine or treatment; some of them affecting the name of systems, and all deriving too much support from credulity or other causes, even among medical men themselves.

Look at what is necessary, in strict reason, to attest the action and value of a new remedy or method of treatment. The identity or exact relation of the cases in which it is employed; — a right estimate of the habits and tempera-ment, moral as well as physical, of the subjects of experi-ment; — allowance for the many modifications depending on dose, combination, quality of the medicine, and time of

* " Id credunt esse experientiam, quando semel vel bis faustam, vel infelicem, in certo morbo a sumpto medicamento annotarunt efficaciam." — *Hoffman.*

use;—due observation of the indirect or secondary, as well
as direct, effects; — and such observation applied, not to
one organ or function alone, but to the many which constitute the material of life. All these things, and yet
more, are essential to the completeness of the testimony.
All can rarely, if ever, be reached; and hence the inevitable imperfections of medicine as a science. But much
more, doubtless, of truth and beneficial result might be
attained, were these difficulties rightly appreciated, and
the fit means of obviating them kept more constantly in
view.*

In no class of human events is the reasoning of "*post
hoc, propter hoc,*" so commonly applied by the world at
large, as in what relates to the symptoms and treatment of
disease. In none is this judgment so frequently both
erroneous and prejudicial. It would seem as if the very
complexity of the conditions necessary to sound evidence,
tended to beget acquiescence in that which is lightest and
most insufficient for truth. The difficulties occurring in
practice from this source are great, and require a right
temper as well as understanding to obviate them.

Nor is there any subject upon which words and phrases,
whether applied to diseases or remedies, exercise a larger
influence. Terms have descended to us, which we can
hardly put aside,—maxims which fetter the understanding,
—and methods of classification, which prevent the better
suggestions of a sound experience. And these are among

---

* Amongst the other difficulties of evidence in such cases must be
noticed the ambiguity of all language as applied to denote and distinguish sensations; an evil familiar to every medical man, and only
to be obviated by watchful experience.

the evils most aggravated by public opinion, ever prone to be governed by names, and particularly in all that concerns the symptoms and treatment of disease. The deeper the interest belonging to the subject, the greater the liability to error.

But in medical doctrine and theory also, there is scarcely less of difficulty from the nature of the evidence concerned. If example were needed to illustrate this, it might be drawn from what relates to the history of fever, whether idiopathic or symptomatic in kind. Here centuries of research, amidst facts of daily occurrence, have yet left some of the most important questions wholly unresolved ; — such is the difficulty of obtaining unequivocal proofs of nature essential to a just theory. The same with respect to the true doctrine of inflammation ; a question which spreads itself, directly or indirectly, over every part of pathology. Here the most various and diligent inquiries long left it uncertain whether there occurred an increased or diminished action of the capillaries of the inflamed part; or in what mere turgescence differs from inflammation. It is only of late years that the improved power and re-fined use of the microscope has given us more assurance as to the nature and succession of these changes; still leaving, however, various points open to future deter-mination.*

The history of contagious diseases furnishes another in-stance not less remarkable. It is the common belief of the

* I allude here especially to Kaltenbrenner's microscopic researches. The frequent revival of controversy on these points among modern writers shows at once their importance, and the incompleteness of the knowledge yet obtained on the subject.

world, and one plausible enough in its first aspect, that the laws of contagion are simple and readily learnt. No mistake can be greater than this. All parts of the subject, even the circumstances most essential to practice, are wrapt up in doubt; and the evidence is of so intricate a kind, and so much disturbed by seeming exceptions, that the best judgments are perpetually at fault upon it. The same remark may be extended to other classes of disease, where time and the most acute observation have hitherto failed to extricate truth from the multitude of conditions present; but where, nevertheless, we have the certainty of relations hitherto undetermined, the fixing of which belongs to future research, and will well repay it in the result.

The observations just made are not less true in relation to the various remedies we employ, even those most familiar, and seemingly simplest in use. The difficulties already noticed as belonging to the evidence of their effects, extend yet further, and more remarkably, to the theory of their action; and our knowledge, though augmented of late years by the wonderful advance of organic Chemistry, can scarcely yet be said to have passed the threshold of this inquiry.

On the other side we are bound to admit, that the recent methods of research in medicine have gained greatly in exactness, and the just appreciation of facts, upon those of any previous period: — a natural effect of increasing exactness in all other branches of science; and, it must be added, of increasing and well directed energy amongst those engaged in the profession. A very especial advantage here has been the application of numerical methods and averages to the history of disease; thereby giving it the same course and certainty of result which belong to statistical inquiry on other subjects. Averages may in some sort be termed the mathematics of medical science. It is obvious, indeed, that the value of inferences thus obtained, depends on the exact estimate of what are the *same facts*, —what merely connected by resemblance or partial analogy. Pathological results, essentially different, may be classed together by inexact observers, or by separate observers under different views. These, however, are errors incident to every human pursuit, and best corrected by numerous and repeated averages. The principle in question is indeed singularly effectual in obviating the difficulties of evidence already noticed; and the success with which it has been employed of late, by many eminent observers, affords assurance of the results that may hereafter be expected from this source. Through medical statistics lies the most secure path into the philosophy of medicine.*

In looking further to the chance of overcoming these difficulties in the future, regard must be had to the principle, now verified in so many cases, that in proportion to

* The inquiries which so greatly distinguish M. Louis as a pathologist, may be noted as eminent examples of this method, which is now pursued with great success by many physicians in our own country. The materials furnished for it, under the new Registration Act, are of the most valuable kind; and the volumes already published give full proof of what will be effected for medical science by such a system, so conducted. The same remark applies to the Statistical Reports of the sickness and mortality in the British army on the different Colonial stations, as presented to parliament, and lately published. Besides many other important results, these Reports correct errors which have long existed as to some particular relations between climate and disease.

the complexity of phenomena, is augmented also the number of relations in which they may be surveyed and made the subjects of experiment.*   The application of this principle to medical science is every day becoming more apparent. Every new path of physical knowledge opened, each single fact discovered, has given guidance more or less direct towards the objects still unattained in physiology and the treatment of disease. The unexpectedness of some of the relations, thus determined and converted to use, is the best augury for further advances in this direction of pursuit.

A due estimate among medical men themselves of the nature of the proofs with which they have to deal is now also more especially needful when the older doctrines of physic and physiology are all undergoing the revision required by modern science; and when new medicinal agents are every day produced upon trial, many of them dangerously active in their effects, many suggested by analogies which need to be verified by the most cautious experience. Hasty and imprudent belief may here become a cause of serious mischief; the wider in its spread, as the minds most prone to this credulity are those most ready also to publish to the world their premature conclusions; and thus to mislead the many who found their own practice upon faith in others; or who seek after novelty, as if this were in itself an incontestable good.

---

* M. Comte, in his " Cours de Philosophie Positive," has defined this as a general law, through which compensation is made for the difficulty or impossibility of giving a mathematical form to certain branches of physics; such particularly as relate to the phenomena of organic bodies.

Here, again, I must advert to a circumstance which renders strict attention to the laws of evidence a matter of peculiar obligation at the present time. This is the tendency, so marked in modern physiology, to carry its researches into the more abstruse questions connected with vitality, the nervous power, and the relations of mental and material phenomena,—inquiries justifiable in themselves, but needing to be fenced round by more than common caution as to testimony, and the conclusions thence derived. Yet here especially it is that such precautions have been disregarded; partly, it may be, from the real difficulty and obscurity of the subject—still more, perhaps, from the incompetency of many of those who have taken it into their hands. For these researches, no longer confined to a few as heretofore, have become the property and pursuit of many who wander merely on the confines of science, believing they are within its pale; and whose speculations on what they see are little checked by collateral knowledge, or by a due estimate of the laws and limits of scientific inquiry. The mystery of the subject is in itself a charm and seduction to the mind. They see, and give attention for the first time, to those wonderful phenomena, which, though inherent in the constitution of man, and in the relations of his mental and corporeal nature, are not familiar to common observation. The feelings are thereby excited even more than the reason; and belief is hurried on, and results accredited, with little care for the sufficiency of proof, or knowledge of the many facts which otherwise explain, or contradict, the conclusion. However earnest the desire for truth, imposture rarely fails to mix itself with inquiries so conducted; and increases the practical evil

which always more or less results from error.   Every philosophical physician is bound to watch over these events
as they pass before him; never refusing inquiry, because
what is put forward is new or strange; but requiring evidence in proportion to the unusual character of the facts;
sifting closely that which is offered, and rejecting all conclusions not founded on this basis.*

* While speaking on the question of evidence as applied to these
subjects, in is impossible not to advert to the fact — a very important
one in the history of the human mind — of the great diversities of
intellectual constitution as to this point.   It is in truth one striking
expression of the difference of the reasoning power, testified on the
most ordinary occasions of life, and very remarkably where the subjects
rise to the character of science.   Locke has well said, " There are
some men of one, some of two syllogisms, and no more ; and others
that can advance but one step further."   The distinction here expressed applies closely to every question of evidence.   One man con-
cludes upon proof, which to another has neither weight nor pertinency.
One mind pursues a subject throughout all its relations;   another
follows but a single line to the result.   Such are these natural dis-
parities, as in many cases to preclude any mutual understanding or
communion of the reasoning power.

A regard to this point seems necessary to explain certain records
of animal magnetism, clairvoyance, lucidity, &c., honestly believed
by many ; which would, if verified by sounder proof, alter all our
views of physical phenomena, of the nature of man, and of the Providence ruling in the world.   The default of just and unexceptionable
evidence which we find here, is still more singularly shown in some
recent works of higher scientific pretension, in which the views and
alleged discoveries of Baron Reichenbach are promulgated; upon faith
in experiments, so entirely wanting in all that gives exactness and
truth to scientific research, that they would hardly be accepted for
results of the greatest antecedent probability.   The most obvious
sources of error are unseen or unprovided for ; even such as vitiate
the experiments made in their first stage of progress.   Yet these
researches are conducted by men of honour and good faith, but wanting in that perception of evidence which is essential to the attainment
of truth.

It must, however, be added, that on questions of medical evidence there may be an excess of scepticism as well as of credulity. Sometimes this occurs in effect of a temperament of mind (not uncommon among thinking men) which is disposed to see all things under doubt and distrust. There are other cases, where the same feeling, not originally present, grows upon the mind of physicians who have been too deeply immersed in the details of practice. The hurried passage from one patient to another precludes that close observation, which alone can justify, except under especial circumstances, the use of new remedies or active methods of treatment. From conscience, as well as convenience, they come to confine themselves to what is safe, or absolutely necessary; and thus is engendered by degrees a distrust of all that lies beyond this limit.

Though such scepticism be less dangerous than a rash and hasty belief, it is manifestly hurtful in practice, and an unjust estimate of medicine as a science; both as it now exists, and as it is capable of being extended and improved. No one can reasonably doubt that we have means in our hands, admitting of being turned to large account of good or ill. Equally unreasonable would it be to distrust the knowledge gained from a faithful experience as to the manner of using these means, and others which may hereafter become known to us, safely and beneficially for the relief of disease. The actual progress of medicine during the last thirty years, in all that regards the principles of the science, as well as the details of practice, is the best testimony for the present, and assurance for the future. As respects the two extremes, noticed above, it is certain that there is a middle course, which men of sound sense will perceive; and to which they alone can steadily adhere, amidst the many difficulties besetting at once the judgment and the conduct of the physician.*

I am the rather led to these remarks on the nature of medical evidence, and the causes moral as well as physical affecting it, looking at the wonderful advances which have been made in all other branches of science; not by the addition of new facts only, but even yet more by new methods and instruments of research, and increasing exactness of details in every point of inquiry. The dissimilarity of the proofs, and the greater difficulty of their certain attainment, must ever keep practical medicine in the rear of other sciences. But its still wider scope of usefulness requires that the distance should be abridged as far as possible; and no occasion be lost, — by improved methods as well as by new facts, by more cautious observation and more exact evidence, — of maintaining its place among the other great objects of human knowledge.

* Laplace happily expresses the middle course here designated: " Egalement éloigné de la crédulité qui fait tout admettre, et de la prévention qui porte à rejeter tout ce qui s'écarte des idées reçues."

CHAP. II.

EFFECTS OF MENTAL ATTENTION ON BODILY ORGANS.

AMONG the various phenomena which attest the influence of the mind on the bodily organs, it is only of late years that sufficient notice has been taken of those peculiar effects which depend on the act of concentrating the attention singly and severally upon them.* The influence of the will on the voluntary organs, and of the passions and emotions of mind upon other parts of the animal economy, have long been the subject of study. Not equally so the influence of the consciousness thus directed by voluntary effort or otherwise to particular organs and parts of the body — a faculty which to a certain extent the mind undoubtedly possesses; and which, though closely or even indissolubly linked with others of its functions, is nevertheless essentially distinct in its nature and results. It may be exercised as a mental act, even

---

* At the time when this chapter was first published (1839), Müller had dwelt more explictly on this subject than any other physiologist; but limiting his considerations chiefly to the effects of attention in augmenting the intensity of ordinary sensations. More recently this class of facts has been carefully and ably examined; partly from their relation to the mesmeric and other analogous phenomena; still further, from their intrinsic interest as a branch of physiological inquiry. In the writings of Dr. Laycock and Dr. Carpenter, and in several articles of the British and Foreign Med. Chirurg. Review, the subject is treated with great ability and under áll its different bearings.

without the suggestion of previous sensation from these
parts; and though in such cases originating in the will, it
produces no true voluntary movements. When, indeed,
the attention is directly excited by impressions from the
bodily organs, it is not always easy to separate the description from that of sensation itself. But we obviously
require another name and definition for that act by which
the consciousness, with or without such excitement, receives, as it were, a local impulse and direction; remains
fixed on one spot with more or less intentness, and for
longer or shorter time; and produces effects not merely
on the sensations thence derived, but seemingly also in
many cases on the physical state and functions of the
parts concerned.

Though the general inquiry into this class of phenomena
has not, until of late, been explicitly made, yet the
familiarity of the effects, and of the language applied to
them — as well as the speculations regarding a vital principle common to physiologists of every age — may be said
to have implied the more material points in question.
Before entering on the subject, however, I must premise
a few words as to this act of mind, which we designate
attention; a term apparently needing no definition, yet
which is open to some difference of interpretation, depending on the different functions, of mind and body, with
which it is associated, or by which it is brought into
action. The phrase of *direction of consciousness* might
often be advantageously substituted for it; but here again
the same explanation is required as to the especial manner
in which the consciousness is thus called into exercise.
Limiting the question, as we do at present, to the effects

on the bodily organs, we have to note the several distinctions between attention directed to any part by express effort of the will — attention solicited by sensations derived from the part, and independent of all volition — and attention suggested or excited by some mental state, having reference to the part, but in which the will is equally unconcerned. These cases, though ever graduating into one another, as is common with all mental phenomena, yet are essentially distinct; and even where scarcely divisible to observation, do still severally modify, more or less, the results in which they concur. The function of the will, exercised in the first case, and only partially, or not at all, in the others, best defines the separation, and has greatest influence on all the phenomena.

For the moment, however, without looking further into the nature of this power, or the distinctions belonging to it, let us take some examples in proof how general such effects are, and how remarkable in their character and influence on the economy of life. Many of these examples may be tested by the experience even of those wholly unused to such researches.* The phenomena are not insulated or partial, but blend themselves with every function of healthy existence; and are often still more striking under conditions of disease. If disguised to common apprehension, this arises, as in so many other cases, rather from their familiarity and habitual occurrence as an

---

* It must be noticed, however, in regard to such experiments, that the act of attention cannot be thus exercised without some effort and habit of mental control. And, further, that the attention directed long and uninterruptedly to the same object, whether of internal or external sense, confuses, impairs, or otherwise alters the sensations, and strains and exhausts the mind itself.

integral part of life, than from any ambiguity as to the facts themselves.

Before specifying particular instances, however, it must be remarked that the term *direction of consciousness*, in its local application to the bodily organs, is to be understood in a general sense. It is rather upon a region, or compound member, of the body, than upon a particular organ or texture, that the attention can be said thus to concentrate itself. The complex physical structure which pervades the whole frame hardly allows other interpretation than this of the act we are describing. There is reason, however, to believe, though it is difficult to define the facts exactly, that different parts or textures are differently affected by the consciousness thus directed to them; either from diversity in the organs themselves, or from some more obscure inequality in the exercise of the power. The parts concerned in voluntary action would seem to be more sensitive to the attention directed to them by voluntary effort than are other parts of the body; though none of the ordinary muscular movements depending on the will follow such direction.

To begin now with the examples which offer themselves in illustration, derived from the voluntary exercise of this faculty.

The effect of attention directed to the heart, and organs of circulation and respiration, is rendered ambiguous from the facility with which these parts are affected by every mental emotion, however slight in degree; and by the difficulty of separating attention, as an act of mind, from the emotional feelings. Yet there is cause to believe the action of the heart often quickened or otherwise disturbed, by the mere centring the consciousness upon it, without any emotion or anxiety. On occasions where its beats are audible, observation will give proof of this — or the physician can very often infer it while feeling the pulse. And where there is liability to irregular pulsation, such action is seemingly brought on, or increased, by the effort of attention, even though no obvious emotion be present. I have reason also to think that hæmorrhage (as in the simple case of epistaxis) is often increased by the same cause; but whether by excitement to the heart's action, or by direct influence on the vessels of the part, cannot easily be decided. Stimulated attention, moreover, will frequently give a local sense of arterial pulsation where not previously felt; and create or augment those singing and rushing noises in the ears, which probably depend on the circulation through the capillary vessels.

The same may be said of the parts concerned in respiration. If this act be expressly made the subject of consciousness, it will be felt to undergo some change; generally to be retarded at first, and afterwards quickened. But the same alterations are so readily produced in the state of respiration by other causes, and even by the effort of earnest attention applied to other parts, that the proof from this source is more equivocal, though the reality of the fact can scarcely be doubted.* The act of yawning may be cited as a part of this function, where the effect of simple attention to the organs is very curiously

* The general effect of any eager act of attention, however directed in checking for a moment the movements of respiration, is a remarkable fact, and connected with many other phenomena of this great function.

shown; producing complex and even violent muscular motions, in which the will and involuntary powers are concurrently engaged. The actions of coughing and sneezing give similar illustrations of the fact; the attention here being generally excited by some local irritation already existing.

A similar concentration of consciousness on the region of the stomach creates in these parts a sense of weight, oppression, or other less definite uneasiness; and whenever the stomach is full appears greatly to disturb the digestion of the food. This portion of the body is well known to be singularly under the influence of all mental emotions; and it is difficult, as we have seen, so far to individualize or simplify the act of attention, as to remove it wholly out of this class. Yet experiment, which every one can make for himself, will show how readily the functions of the stomach may be altered and disturbed from this cause. The sensation of an uneasy weight is often almost immediate; and this is kept up, or augmented, if the mental act be continued. The symptoms of the dyspeptic patient are doubtless much aggravated by the constant and earnest direction of his mind to the digestive organs, and the functions going on in them. Feelings of nausea may be produced, or greatly increased, in this way; and are often suddenly relieved by the attention being directed to other objects. The proofs of this are frequent and familiar, especially in the incidents of sea-sickness, which afford much curious illustration of the matter before us.

All parts of the alimentary canal are probably subject, though more obscurely, to the same influence. Sensations occur of which we were not before conscious; and the actions of the lower bowel in particular, where voluntary and involuntary functions are combined, are obviously excited and quickened by this cause. Such also, and even more remarkably, is the case with the bladder. Without any direct need from repletion, it is always more or less solicited to act, by the attention directed to it—this sensation, even when painful in degree, ceasing wholly for a time if the mind be diverted to other objects. The generative organs furnish illustrations of similar kind, and to the same effect.

The organs of articulation and deglutition are variously subject to the same influence. The act of swallowing, for instance, becomes manifestly embarrassed, and is made more difficult, by the attention fixed upon it when the morsel to be swallowed comes into contact with the part. This effect depends in part, probably, on the conjunction of voluntary and involuntary action in the same function; a combination always producing very complex and curious phenomena, the right analysis of which give us guidance to many most important results, both in physiology and pathology.

The act of articulation, in its various forms, is as obviously subject to the influence we are describing; and especially where there exists already some impediment to the function. This is curiously illustrated in many cases of stammering; and also in paralytic cases, where the organs of speech are affected by the disease.

The power which this stimulated attention to particular parts of the body has in altering, as well the sensations thence derived, as also even their functional state, may be instanced in many other ways. The salivary glands, for example, are manifestly affected in their secretion; an organ, it may be remarked, singularly susceptible of being affected instantly by mental emotions.* We have reason from observation to believe that the secretion of milk from the mammæ, — an organ also very susceptible, — is often altered by the act of attention alone.   The feelings produced in the tongue in like way are peculiar and well marked; and in the teeth and gums the sensations brought on may rise even into pain, especially if the attention be excited by some irritation already present.

We may reasonably refer to the same principle some of the alleged facts in Homœopathy; such as the long train of symptoms, sometimes amounting to hundreds, which are catalogued as proceeding from infinitesimally small quantities of substances, inert or insignificant in other manner of use.   The attention urged to seek for local sensations has no difficulty in finding them.   They generate one another; and are often, as we shall afterwards see, excited by the mere expectation of their occurrence.†

---

* May not the influence of mental emotions on the stomach depend in part in the changes thereby produced on the secreting glands of this organ? We have evidence to this effect in the various glands, connected with the digestive organs, which are more immediately within our observation.

† The manner in which these alleged symptoms are collected and registered by Homœopathists, must be regarded as a glaring instance of the want of due understanding of evidence, referred to in the preceding chapter.   Apart from the intrinsic improbability of the same agent, in doses inappreciably minute, producing effects on numerous parts wholly different in structure and function, we find the proofs (even as they come from the founder of the doctrine) to consist principally in the simple assertion of the subjects of experi-

The instances hitherto given belong chiefly to the organs of internal function ; but the effects of attention concentrated on the immediate organs of sense are more familiar to us, and of great importance in our constitution. Though the inference is ambiguous, as may well happen from the nature of the actions concerned, we have cause to suppose that physical changes, whatever their nature, are induced on the organs; altering, and for the most part augmenting, the intensity of the sensations they convey. No one can direct his consciousness to the organs of seeing, hearing, or even of taste, without becoming aware of some changes in their state, from the mind thus by effort applied to them. It is even possible, as learnt by experiment, to give a different intensity to the impressions received from one or other eye, or ear, by the agency of the mind severally upon these parts. And explanation of the improvement of the senses by exercise may readily be found in the habitual repetition of this mental action, and its effects on the physical condition of the organs — in conformity with the more general law, that any frequently repeated action of a part invites more of blood and nervous power into it; adding, unless there be excess of action, to its power and capacity.

Carrying on the inquiry from these organs of sense to the sensorium itself, we find our research speedily lost in obscurity, its very conditions rendering vain every hope of satisfactory result. All that can be said is, that the attention

ment; unchecked, as far as we can see, by any regard to the phenomena now before us, though so absolutely essential to the truth of all conclusions thus obtained.

by an effort of will concentrated upon the seat of the brain, creates certain vague feelings of tension and uneasiness, caused possibly by some change in the circulation of the part; though it may be an effect, however difficult to conceive, on the nervous system itself. Persistence in this effort, which is seldom indeed possible beyond a short time, produces results of much more complex nature, and scarcely to be defined by the terms of common language. It is in fact the case of the mind turned inwards upon the organs which most closely minister to its own operations; and by this reflex act, disturbing the latter in every part;—a circumstance I do not find to have been duly noticed, instructive though it is in regard to some of the most abstruse relations of our mental existence.

One curious phenomenon may perhaps be noticed here, though probably connected more with the internal cerebral organisation of the senses, than with any part of the intellectual functions. This is, the influence of attention directed inwards upon those images or repetitions of objects of sense, which, even in the waking state, are perpetually generated within the sensorium; independently of all direct impressions from without, though often immediately consequent upon them. Occasionally, these *subjective images* (to borrow a German term for this obscure and difficult subject) acquire such morbid intensity, as to usurp powerfully upon the reason — a fact of which some singular examples will be found in a succeeding Chapter (on Dreaming, Insanity, &c.). But taking them in their more simple and common occurrence,—as, for instance, in the changeable coloured spectra which appear when the eyes are closed, after gazing on a bright luminous object; or the image, under like circumstances, of a window perfectly pictured to this inward vision — the influence of the attention, directed or suspended, is as well manifested in regard to these images as towards those directly derived from objects without. The Daguerrotype picture of the window (a description well admissible here) may wholly disappear for a short time; and then be recalled, though less vividly, by the attention again directed to it.* It is difficult to affirm absolutely that these cases are the same in kind, or that they graduate into those more remote images, which traverse the sensorium, wholly dissociated from any present sensation. The subject is very obscure, and blends itself with the most abstruse points of metaphysical inquiry. But there is strong presumption, from analogy, for such relation; and the act of mental attention associates itself with and modifies each class of phenomena.

I have not yet adverted, except in general terms, to the effects of attention on those parts of the body with which muscular actions and the sense of touch are more intimately connected. This, however, is a very interesting part of the subject; not merely as illustrating it in many important points; but, yet further, in relation to various striking phenomena, which, without such principle applied to their explanation, might well be deemed anomalies in the course and condition of human life. The observations here, moreover, admit of being more widely varied

* I have often succeeded (for these are experiments which every man may make for himself) in bringing back this image of the window, after the eyes had been opened for a moment and again closed; with care, however, that the intervening objects of vision should present no strong contrast of light and shade.

and methodised by experiment, and afford clearer inferences than those made on internal organs.   One limb,
for instance, or even a single finger, or a portion of the
sentient surface of the body, can be taken for observation,
and the results tested and checked by means wholly
independent of the subject of experiment; a point often
very important to the truth of the result.

We have here, as in other parts of the inquiry, to look
to the respective cases of attention directed by express
volition, or suggested by some outward cause acting on
the mind.   In the former and more simple case, if a limb
be taken for experiment, a peculiar sense of weight, with
a vibratory tingling, or sensations· approaching to cramp,
are produced by the consciousness concentrated upon it.
It is difficult to describe by words feelings of this nature,
evanescent or changing at each moment, and different,
doubtless, in different persons: but probably the closest
resemblance is to those produced in ordinary cases by
muscular fatigue, or stagnant circulation through the limb.
There is reason, indeed, to suppose that the muscular structure is actually affected in these cases, and frequently even
by particular conditions of movement, though not volitional
in kind; as instanced in the old experiments with the
Divining Rod, and others analogous in kind, but of more
recent date. *   It would seem that certain tremulous

---

* This science of the Divining Rod, or Rabdomancy, boasting a high
descent, and putting forward a large array of proofs, had for a long period
numerous professors and believers in every part of Europe, though now
almost wholly displaced by better evidence, or other fashions of belief.
I may briefly allude here to some experiments made under my own
eyes at Milan, by Amoretti, the last professor and writer, as far as I

motions — it may be the first stage of true muscular contraction — occur in these cases; capable, especially where
expectation is blended with the act of attention, of communicating movement to objects with which the muscles
are in contact; and even, unconsciously, of rendering such
movement conformable in direction to the expectation entertained. Some interesting experiments were made by
Chevreul, several years ago, with results of this character.
But whatever the nature of the effect on muscular structure or action, no doubt can exist as to the occurrence of
new and specific sensations from the attention directed in
the manner described.*

know, on the mystery of the *Verga Divinatoria* (*Amoretti, sulla Scienza
della Raddomanzia*). In these experiments, as I witnessed them, a
main point was to show that the divining rod (a fork or double branch
of hazel), grasped firmly at each end, tended strongly to move and revolve
in the proximity of certain metals, water, &c., requiring more or less
force to prevent it. The trials had various results with different persons. When most successful, I could, on close inspection, perceive
certain slight movements and contractions of the muscles of the thumb,
though those holding the stick were not conscious of this. I, myself,
though attentive to prevent muscular action, had difficulty in doing
so entirely; but this difficulty was the same when the objects supposed to compel the rotation of the rod were removed. The so-named
rod itself was of form and texture most prone to easy rotation; and
the manner directed for holding it such, as to make the very firmness
of the grasp conducive to the effect.

* My attention was first drawn to this point very many years ago,
when witnessing some Mesmeric experiments of the late Mr. Chenevix;
more simple and unpretending than those of our own time, but applied
to the same class of subjects, and similarly conducted as to the manner
of proof. These experiments, made with two young girls, were to the
effect of inducing various sensations—heat, weight, or inability of
motion—in any limb to which the attention was expressly solicited by
Mesmeric means applied, and by the questions asked. The proof

Or, again, if a portion of the surface of the body be made the subject of this influence, sensations of heat or cold on the skin, or other more vague feelings of tightness or tingling, are readily created, hardly definite enough for description, but sufficiently so for proof. In that state of skin, however produced, of which itching is a symptom, the attention directed upon any particular part will very often bring this sensation immediately to it. Such cases as these, where it is difficult to prove more than a change or increase of feeling in the parts affected, may appear ambiguous in evidence. But that some real alteration takes place, either in their nervous condition or circulation, or both, is probable from the distinct evidence of this in other instances of the mental consciousness thus locally directed.

These instances, to which we now come, merit the closest observation. They involve, not mere attention directed by a simple act of will, but attention to parts and functions of the body suggested or forcibly excited by impressions on the mind itself — separate from and only partially controlled by the will — and producing effects, both of sensation and motion, far more remarkable than those hitherto described. Such impressions on the mind

here as to the real nature of the causes concerned was afforded by the repetition of the experiments, at my request, with the *show* of the same means applied' (a mere slip of paper placed by the Mesmeriser upon the limb), but with nothing actually done. The effect was precisely the same as before in the description of sensations produced; and this result was obtained repeatedly, with little variation. I was led at the time, and often since, to make the trial on myself; and always with sensations more or less resembling those described above, when sufficient effort was made to *localise* the attention, and keep it fixedly on the point designed.

may arise either from outward objects, through the senses ; or from changes in the sensorium itself. But for the right understanding of their nature and effects, it is needful to premise a few remarks on this great function of the will, which is so deeply engaged in all these various acts of life, yet at the same time checkèd and controlled on every side by the automatic and material parts of our nature.

The struggle, for such it may often be termed, between voluntary and involuntary acts — between the intellectual and automatic functions—is, in truth, a dominant fact in the mental constitution of man ; one upon which all the phenomena, both of mind and body, closely depend at every instant of life. In using the term *struggle*, however, let it be added that there is no provision of our nature which better illustrates the wisdom and prescience to which we owe our being. Man might have been created with larger powers than he has—but under the limitation manifestly designed by his Creator, we must ever admire that wonderful adaptation, by which faculties, different in nature, and often opposed in action, do yet concur and harmonise in general results ; giving order and stability to all the complex functions of life, and admitting of increase of power to those of the highest kind by their due and sufficient exercise. We might have been constituted, so as to regulate by will those of our actions which are now automatic or instinctive. Were these functions suddenly committed to us, disorder and death would speedily ensue.

The balance between these powers is, however, liable to perpetual fluctuations during life ; in many cases from natural causes, such as sleep, in its various states of kind and degree — in other cases from morbid conditions of the

body, and particularly of the nervous system—in other instances, again, from emotions or affections, however generated, of the mind itself. All these several causes, which
might be exemplified by innumerable details, alter and
disturb more or less the action of the will; in some cases
rendering it feeble and uncertain, in others apparently for
a time abolishing it altogether. The study of these several
gradations of change ; of the causes producing them ; of
their effect in giving temporary predominance to the more
automatic parts of our being; and of the peculiar temperaments most liable to be thus affected, is perhaps the most
instructing part of human physiology, and most largely illustrative of the mental and bodily relations of man. Every
moment of life furnishes examples — difficult, it may be, of
analysis in ordinary cases — but in others, and these of
common occurrence, strikingly marked by the disparity
and struggle of the two powers.

In speaking of the automatic, however, as opposed to
the voluntary power, we must not limit the former to what
are commonly termed the parts and functions of organic
life, — those which depend on the spinal and ganglionic
systems, and the direct and reflex actions therewith connected. We can hardly apply any other term to those
states of the sensorial organs, in which there is the loss,
partially or completely, of voluntary power over the ideas,
images, or creations which successively traverse the mind ;
as well as of the influence of the will over the voluntary
muscles of the body. The rational governance of these
acts is enfeebled or gone; and the influence of organic or
material causes comes in, producing those vague and inconsequent trains of thought and imagery, which we have

just denoted as strongly expressed in the states of sleep and disease; but which are of constant occurrence, in one degree or another, in all the passages of life. In many re-markable cases the ordinary perceptions from the senses are wholly disturbed and perverted by the condition of the sensorium receiving them. Muscular motions occur from other causes than volition; and past images and memories rise up unbidden to perplex both sensations and acts by mingling with them, without control or direction of the rational will.

We can hardly go further in deciphering this most obscure part of our nature, present though its effects ever are to our consciousness. But these effects are too rapid in sequence, the changes in the power and direction of the will too frequent and transient, to be submitted to analysis. We recognise the main fact of its limitation by the auto-matic parts of our structure; we see and feel it to be variously controlled by impressions from without and states of mind within; we observe the influences of these several causes in creating habits of action, mental as well as bodily, in which the power of the will is so far lost that they become almost like the instincts of inferior life.* In

---

* Though habits contracted in life often assume the character of instincts, in their persistence, regularity, and separation from volun-tary control; yet must we regard them, in their origin and nature, as essentially distinct principles of action. In a subsequent chapter, especially directed to the topic of instincts and habits, will be found some more detailed observations on this most interesting portion of physiology. It is a subject which we cannot too closely study for our better comprehension of the whole; there being in effect no part of the history or philosophy of life with which it is not intimately con-cerned.

the ensuing chapters of this volume will be found farther
illustration of these phenomena, in their relations to various
conditions, natural or morbid, of the life of man ; and the
subject of that immediately following (Chap. III.) will,
I think, furnish some suggestions as to the principle in our
constitution on which these remarkable changes depend.
In the succeeding chapters on Sleep, Dreaming, Insanity,
&c., instances will be given, which well illustrate the
different stages of insubordination to the will in functions
naturally submitted to its influence ; and furnish explanation of those singular states of reverie, trance, hysteria,
spectral vision, catalepsy, &c., which express the conflicts
and changes thus taking place.

It is this class of cases we have to notice, in reverting to
the more immediate subject before us. Here the attention,
no longer guided,—or if at all, partially and interruptedly,
— by the rational will, becomes submitted to the vague
and almost automatic conditions of the sensorium just
described. The actions upon it from without, and the
reflected acts and movements thereby induced, form a very
extraordinary page in the history of the human mind. It
is here, in fact, that we must look for explanation of those
strange results in Animal Magnetism, Electrobiology, &c.,
which have served so greatly to perplex all ordinary
observers, and even some who come better prepared for the
scrutiny of such phenomena. Without referring in detail
to things often described and very generally known, I
will at once point out the questions which concern us in
the present inquiry ; and which govern, in truth, every
other question and argument in relation to the topics just
mentioned. Are these phenomena—admitted by all to be

singular and striking — derived from a peculiar agent or influence, transmitted from one human body to another by certain modes of communication? Or are they the effects of various external excitements on the sensorium and nervous system of persons of a peculiar temperament, analogous in nature and origin to phenomena with which we are more familiar in sleep, trance, hysteria, and other forms of cerebral or nervous disorder?

These questions, involving the very reality of the Mesmeric theory, must ever be kept before us in all observation or reasoning on the subject. It is singularly important that this should be done wherever experiment is concerned; inasmuch as they suggest those particular tests which are essential to complete evidence, but which have been, for the most part, unaccountably neglected. In putting these questions, moreover, we indicate the absolute need, for the right prosecution of this inquiry, of familiarity with the natural phenomena of health and disease just adverted to. Without this knowledge, and without the just perception of what constitutes scientific evidence, we might as well be gazing on the feats of a conjuror at a public exhibition, as on those of animal magnetism in similar assemblies.

Another point in this question, not sufficiently kept in mind, is the vast distinction between the two classes of Mesmeric phenomena, — sleep, reverie, trance, and certain acts arising from them, — and the miraculous assumption of clairvoyance, prophecy, and other powers, superseding all the physical laws of time and space of which we have any knowledge. These things are presented to us as parts of the same phenomenon, and produced by the same mani-

pulations or personal contact. But they are in truth of
very different nature, and totally incommensurate with
each other. There is less distinction between the intellect
of an infant and that of Bacon, Newton, or Laplace, than
between the conditions thus brought into pretended connexion. If the miraculous powers in question, for they
admit no other name, be proffered to our belief, it must be
upon evidence far more searching and stringent than is
needed to verify those other conditions, which are so
closely allied to the ordinary changes in health and disease.
It is unnecessary to dilate on the importance of a distinction which every man of understanding will admit and
appreciate.

Another frequent error of belief it is also important to
remove. The phenomena which have been produced under
the name of Electrobiology, have manifestly close rela-
tionship to those of Mesmerism, and are connected by
common opinion with the same mysterious cause. Yet
this remarkable class of facts does in fact contradict what
we have seen to be the main assumption of the Mesmerists; — that, namely, of a bodily influence of A. upon B.,
by which the latter is brought into what could only be
considered a new state of existence; mental as well as
bodily, active as well as passive. The results exhibited by
the Biologists—analogous in kind and equally striking—
are not alleged to proceed from any such mysterious
agency; but come before us fairly as the very curious
effect of excitement of various kinds upon certain peculiar
temperaments; and, as such, well illustrate some of the
topics under discussion in this chapter, and are reciprocally

illustrated by them. These relations have been ably examined and commented upon ; and proof given that all the more credible results of animal magnetism (and the experiments of Baron Reichenbach come under the same class) may be obtained from a more natural source than that in which Mesmerists profess to believe.

A further connexion still remains to be noted between these questions and the general subject before us. In speaking of the frequent struggle between the voluntary and automatic parts of our nature, and of the singular impairment or loss of voluntary power, and change in other mental faculties from certain impressions on the sensorium, we alluded to the remarkable diversity in different temperaments, as respects their liability to these changes. Much more might be said on this point, and much, in truth, is suggested by the phenomena to which we are now adverting. Amongst the main facts in Mesmerism, and the agencies having kindred with it, the following are especially to be noted. First, the vast difference in the proneness of different persons to be thus affected. Secondly, the small comparative number who are liable at all. Thirdly, the very large proportion of females among the number so acted upon. Taking, for better illustration, the opposite extremes of liability, it becomes, in fact, the distinction between those wholly insusceptible of such influence, and others who are affected at any instant; and with susceptibility ever increasing by frequency of repetition. The consideration of these extreme cases, as well as of the gradations between them, is a matter of much interest, as illustrating the varieties of human temperament; and both in this and other points comes closely

D

in connexion with our subject. Adopting the terms in pathological use, we may affirm that the nervous or hysterical temperament is that most prone to be thus acted upon; and that in the extreme cases of such susceptibility this idiosyncrasy touches closely on epilepsy, catalepsy, or other forms of cerebral disorder. It may safely be stated, that of those most affected by Mesmeric means, or by the Odyle of Reichenbach, nine out of ten are females, or youths of the same nervous temperament; and that of the former, the majority are under 25 years of age.*

Applying these facts to the more mysterious exhibitions

---

* I believe that the records of these cases, as published in England, France, and Germany, will, if duly examined, fully bear out this statement. The subjects of those of Baron Reichenbach's experiments upon which he mainly grounds his conclusions and theory, were all females under thirty; and all of them admitted to have some peculiarity of nervous constitution or habit, such as catalepsy, paralysis, somnambulism, or spasmodic affections; a point obviously of much moment to the evidence, though unaccountably neglected in this light.

In connexion with this subject it is needful to refer, however slightly, to a class of cases, familiar more or less to every medical man, where this peculiar temperament, especially in young girls, begets a habit and intense desire of imposture, which may well be deemed a sort of moral insanity. My own practice has furnished me with several such instances; hardly credible in their details, from the artifices displayed and the extraordinary bodily sufferings undergone, to substantiate what was usually but an idle and unmeaning fraud. It cannot be doubted that cases of this kind have mingled themselves with the history of Animal Magnetism, both in our own country and elsewhere; and it is especially needful to keep this in mind when called upon to credit that higher pretension of powers which contravene all experience and every recognised physical law.

A passage of Lord Bacon, closely applying to this subject, will be remembered by many: — "Delight in deceiving and aptness to be deceived, imposture and credulity, although they appear to be of a diverse nature, yet certainly they do for the most part concur." — *On the Advancement of Learning*.

of this influence, they cogently suggest the question, how it can happen that such manifestations of new and exalted power — the knowledge of events far distant in space and time—the instant recognition, without inquiry, of the seat and nature of internal disease and of the befitting treatment—vision, or that perception which is equivalent to it, through other organs than the eyes, &c. — how it happens, I say, that faculties so marvellous should be given to those of feeble, vague, or distempered mind, and wholly denied to men of the highest mental energy and intellectual powers?—given, moreover, by persons who themselves possess none of the faculties which they thus miraculously bestow? This question, though stated merely as such, is in effect pregnant with argument; and deserves to be well weighed by all who incline to this separate and more mysterious part of Mesmeric belief.

I have dwelt so far upon this particular topic, both from the various illustrations it affords to our present subject, and also because the phenomena alluded to are themselves in this connexion best illustrated and explained. The influence of attention, as an act of mind voluntary or involuntary, upon the bodily organs, admits, however, of yet further exemplification. The many instances hitherto given are chiefly derived from what may be deemed the healthy or normal state. Disease and disordered functions furnish examples equally numerous and remarkable; a few of which it will be desirable to notice, in completion of the inquiry. They will doubtless suggest many others to the recollection of every intelligent practitioner.

To the cure of the dyspeptic I have already sufficiently alluded in illustration. Closely akin to this is the disorder

of the hypochondriac, some of the most singular perversions
of which admit of the same explanation. Here the
patient, in fixing his consciousness with morbid intentness
on different organs, creates not merely disordered sensations, but often, also, disordered actions in them. There
may be palpitation of the heart, hurried or choked respiration, flatulence, and other distress of stomach, irritation of
the bladder, vague neuralgic pains; all arising from this
morbid direction of attention to the organs in question.
It is certain that many of the secretions are immediately
affected by emotions of mind; and the same effect appears
to arise from anxious and sustained attention to the parts
concerned in these functions.

In chorea, hysteria, and other diseases where disordered
nervous actions occur, the same principle is more or less
involved; but without any such distinct intervention of
the consciousness and will, as in most of the examples
already cited. Yet in hysteria, and generally in what has
been called the hysteric temperament, the instances are
frequent of attacks being brought on by the mere expectation of them, or, occasionally, even by a sort of *morbid
solicitation* of the organs to these singular actions. Of the
latter facts medical experience furnishes numerous examples; and here, again, we trace to their probable origin
many of the more remarkable incidents of animal magnetism. The influence upon the external organs of what has
been called *expectant attention* belongs especially to this
temperament; and though in some part a natural phenomenon, yet it is brought into a degree of activity in certain habits, and under certain excitements, which gives it
the character of a morbid state, and evolves many remark-

able results. The sensation, or action, or suspension of power of action, may all be produced by the excited expectation created at the moment of these several effects; an influence very strikingly exhibited in the biological experiments to which we have already referred.*

Taking a more simple and familiar instance to the same effect, if immediately after an attack of cramp the attention be kept fixed on the limb so affected, a tendency will be felt to renewal of the spasms, and sometimes they will actually recur from this excitement to the part.

Closely connected with this morbid influence of attention is the effect of simple *imitation* in producing various excited or disordered states of body. The natural act of yawning has already been mentioned. An analogous fact occurs among asthmatic patients, in many of whom I have seen a certain degree of the disorder brought on by seeing others suffering under it. Cough, and other spasmodic actions, are known to be readily excited in similar way. And, again, in the very remarkable disorder of chorea (*St. Vitus's Dance*), where the vague and violent muscular actions are not only involuntary, but almost detached from consciousness, it is a familiar fact that others are often attacked with the same disorder in effect of imitation alone; rendering it necessary to separate the patient from those having a similar nervous temperament and liability to spasmodic

* It is difficult for any one who has not seen these experiments to conceive the full amount of this influence in annulling the will for a time, and in many cases substituting involuntary action for it. Here, however, the proportion of persons fully *sensitive* to the influence is not more than one in ten or twelve — analogous in this to animal magnetism, as might be expected from the close connexion of the pheno‚ mena in their origin and manifestation.

affections. It is obvious that persons of this temperament
are peculiarly unfitted to afford any just evidence in
experiments where external influence is concerned; a
point upon which I have already commented in reference
to the frequent use of them in such researches.

Another very singular case is that of an expected
impression on some part of the body producing, before
actually made, sympathetic sensations or movements in
other parts which are wont to be affected by such impressions.   An example occurs to me at this time of a person,
in whom the mere expectation of any hard pressure of
the hand, or sudden jar of the body, instantly creates uneasiness, approaching to momentary pain, in the perinœum ;
this particular effect, in greater degree, invariably following
actual jar or pressure.   Such instances, while involving
other curious points in physiology, illustrate the dependence of these morbid sympathies and acts of imitation on
the more general principle which forms the subject of the
present chapter.

If now, dispensing with other examples, we recur for a
moment to the elementary view of this principle with
which we set out, our first impression will be, that of its
close connexion and co-ordination with every part of our
existence, mental and bodily, intellectual and moral, under
the conditions of health and disease.   The agency in
question is in truth so incorporated with us,—so integral a
part of the mind in its relation to the bodily organs, as
well as the whole class of mental emotions,—that it is
difficult to make language subserve to its description, or
to the points which need discrimination in its theory.   The

point especially meriting regard is the evidence afforded, that the physical state or function of a part is actually altered from this cause, and not the mental perception only. As far as I am aware, the subject has not been sufficiently examined under this view; though in the various forms which the theory of a vital principle has taken, we have proof of the influence of these facts upon the course of speculation.*

We have still one point in this inquiry remaining for discussion; the solution of which, could it be obtained, would do more than anything besides to remove those ambiguities, both of language and thought, which, as we have seen, crowd round every part of the subject. This is the question, whether any step of physical explanation can be made towards the phenomena? whether that transference of consciousness by volition to particular parts,

---

* The *Archæus* of Van Helmont, and the *Anima* of Stahl (as well as the Πνευματα of Galen and earlier writers), have reference to the agency which is the subject of this chapter. It is obvious that each author sought by such phrases to express an active immaterial principle, producing and controlling the actions of the system, by an operation neither chemical nor mechanical, but in fact identical with life itself. It was the need and effort to find something intervening between mind and body, — some middle agency that might give a show of explanation of the actions of the former upon the latter, — which suggested these terms, and gave a sort of reality to them. In sound reasoning, it is plain that we acquire only new names by their adoption, and no increase of real knowledge.

" There is a connexion of the living principle in the powers of one part with those of another, which may be called a species of intelligence." This is a happy expression of John Hunter, applicable here, and to many other questions in this part of physiology. — *Croonian Lecture on Muscular Motion.*

which we have called attention of mind, takes place through some branch of the nervous system, as volitions are conveyed to the muscular organs? or whether, in default of evidence to this effect, our inquiries must end as they begun, by simply recognising such relation of the sensorium to the bodily organs, as one expression of the individuality of the whole being?

There is one consideration, principally, which makes it highly probable that a direct function of the nerves is concerned in the results before us. This is the fact (a very important one in physiology) that the peculiar relation of the mind to the bodily organs of which we are treating is not alike or equal in degree to all parts; but that it seems to exist for each in some direct proportion to its nervous sensibility, or perhaps also to its vascularity in the healthy state: these two conditions being generally in close relation to each other. And, further, it may be added, in confirmation of this view, that the attention, strongly concentrated on one part, totally precludes for the moment any similar effort being directed to another; in dependence on a law we shall have occasion in the next chapter to illustrate. Admitting these circumstances as founded on observation, they lead directly to the inference that the nerves are in some manner excited by the act of attention, and that all particular and local effects on the body depend on their agency; with a secondary influence from changes in the circulation of the parts, where these effects severally occur.

Upon this conclusion, however, rises another question equally difficult, viz. with what other function of the nerves this action is most closely allied, and through what class of nerves it is carried on ? Those of voluntary motion can scarcely be admitted, seeing that motion in this sense is no part of the effect, and that the influence extends to parts over which we have little or no voluntary power. The only employment of will here is in giving this partial direction to the consciousness. If, on the other hand, we suppose the nerves of sensation concerned, we must admit two several actions in opposite direction along the same tract of nerve ; a condition of which, though not disproved, we have no well-assured evidence. In neither of these functions, therefore, nor in the nerves ministering to them, can we find any certain explanation of the phenomenon before us, though it has various and close relation to both, as they mutually have to each other.

In considering this intricate subject, it is impossible not to advert again to the connexion between attention, as a state of mind, and the whole class of mental emotions ; a relation the more important to be noticed, because it is testified to us by many similar effects of both on the bodily organs, and may afford therefore some presumption that the same nervous agency is concerned in each case. An examination of individual consciousness will afford the best proof as to this relation. The difficulty in following it out, and that which makes it obviously needful to discriminate between the two cases, is the explicit power of the will in directing the attention of mind to particular parts. A faculty exists here distinct from mental emotion, though variously complicated with it ; and especially in those instances where the attention is strongly excited by sensations derived from any organ. As a power, it is equally definite as that by which we change or give direction to the trains of thought, and indeed closely allied to it in many respects.

Reverting to the question, whether there be any especial nervous action, by which we direct the attention of mind to different parts of the body — and if any, what are the nerves engaged in that function ? — the admission must at once be made, that we are not furnished with any present means to solve the difficulty. I have tried to obtain evidence in cases where there was palsy of a limb, affecting either the nerves of sensation, or those of voluntary motion. But though some of the results seemed to show loss or enfeeblement of the power, especially in the former cases, there was too much ambiguity from other sources to admit of other inference than that already stated, as to these nerves. Any impairment of the power, under paralysis of the sentient nerves, cannot be received as expressing more than the want of the ordinary reflex action upon the sensorium through this channel.

The effect upon the circulation of a part from the consciousness suddenly directed and fixed upon it, is often so obvious and immediate, that we might, perhaps, suppose the nerves belonging appropriately to the vascular system to be engaged in producing them. But this is an influence so obscure in itself, and which we are so unprovided with any further means of substantiating by proof, that it is not worth while to speculate upon it. In truth, the difficulty here is one which extends largely over all that relates to the functions of the nervous system. Scarcely yet have all its parts been thoroughly defined in reference to the two great functions of sensation and volition ; while the ganglionic system and the nerves of organic life are still only partially known to us in their proper action, and still more obscurely in their intricate connexions with the various powers of animal life. On this subject I shall have to speak further in a future chapter.*

I must not quit this topic, however, without adverting to the important view regarding reflex actions of the brain, analogous to those of the medulla spinalis, propounded by Dr. Laycock some years ago. This view, which has close relation to all the phenomena we have been recording, merits, in every way, further illustration and research; and particularly in reference to the whole theory of habits and instinctive actions. It holds out, indeed, no solution to the physiological question just stated; but, if well founded, advances us a step nearer to such solution. †

The physiological facts treated of in the present chapter have close relation to the faculty the mind possesses of withdrawing itself wholly or partially from objects of sense which yet physically impress the external organs in the same way as when fully perceived, shifting itself to other sensations or to trains of internal thought, sometimes by direct effort of the will sometimes, in effect of causes with which the will has no concern. Every moment of life affords instances in illustration of this. We live, it

---

* See the last chapter of this volume.

† Dr. Laycock's paper, expounding this view, was read to the Medical Section of the British Association, at York, in 1844. Though coming as a sort of supplement to the doctrine of reflex actions of the medulla spinalis, which we owe to the valuable labours of Dr. Marshall Hall, it cannot from its nature admit of the same amount of evidence or certainty of conclusion

may be said, in a series of acts or states, each involving the exercise of some particular faculty or sense, to the exclusion, more or less, of others; but all so blended by instant sequence, and in such subordination to the identity of the being, that we are speedily at fault in seeking to decide or minutely analyse the succession. This topic, very closely associated in every way with that now before us, will form the especial subject of the ensuing chapter. In discussing it, I shall have occasion to advert in detail to the faculty the mind possesses of separating and arranging anew for its own perception objects equally and simultaneously present to the organs of sense — a power upon which our intellectual existence largely depends, and which has not, I think, received all the notice which its importance deserves.

Every instance of this nature, and all the topics indeed of this chapter, are subordinate to the great inquiry regarding the relation of consciousness and volition in the sentient being, to those functions of the different organs of sense, which connect this being with its own bodily organisation and with the world without. This, in truth, is the fundamental mystery of animal life. The difficulty, as well as importance of the questions it involves, increase as we rise from the simpler forms of existence to those where the intellectual and moral faculties are more fully developed. In man these phenomena take their most complex character; and the ever changing relation of individual consciousness in the sentient unity, to the different bodily and mental actions which form the totality of life, illustrates best, though it may not explain, the endless varieties and seeming anomalies of human existence. Instincts, habits, insanity, dreaming, somnambulism, and trance, all come within the scope of this principle; which points out, moreover, connexions among them, not equally to be understood in any other mode of viewing the subject. *

* I had once intended to bring into this chapter the consideration of the influence of the mental passions and emotions on the bodily economy, as being thus closely connected with its subject. But the topic is so wide in itself, and associated with so many others in metaphysical and moral philosophy, that I have judged it better not to embarrass by this addition an argument already so much extended.

CHAP. III.

ON MENTAL CONSCIOUSNESS, IN ITS RELATION TO TIME AND SUCCESSION.

THE phenomena alluded to at the close of the last chapter, though forming the very staple of our mental existence, and familiar to us, more or less, in every act of life, are yet little recognised, or made the subject of examination.* This familiarity, indeed, as in many kindred cases, disguises what is so wonderful in them, when closely scrutinised. Ever living in a series of mental states or acts, we become regardless of the manner of change and sequence, and of the relation of these successive states to the great element of time, which pervades the whole. Some object of sense is before the mind to the momentary exclusion of others; thought follows such perception, excluding for a time all objects of external sense; remembrances crowd upon thought, and furnish it with ever-changing subjects;

---

* So closely is the subject of this chapter connected with that of the last, that I have had some hesitation which to place first in the volume. It is one of the many instances we shall have to note, showing how all the phenomena of life and mind graduate into one another; making it often more difficult to dissever and distinguish than to combine the facts that come before us.

passions and emotions are blended in the same current, but equally under constant change and succession. Volition in some cases governs and guides the sequence; and selects, as it were, the objects of present perception and thought. At other times the mind seems as if submitted to the changes of state, which come upon it unbidden and despite the will.

The deep interest of the questions here suggested will at once be admitted, as well as the legitimate nature of the inquiries. Though there is but a single channel through which it may be pursued, yet this is open to every one in his individual consciousness. The faculty, or principle, described under this name, can alone furnish us with those elementary facts which lie at the bottom of all mental philosophy, under whatever name propounded.

What, then, is this consciousness? Scarcely can we render the conception of it clearer by definition, or describe what is inseparable from our existence and identity of being. Language here, as so often elsewhere, fails in meeting the emergency; and the very simplicity of the fact tends to make it less obvious to common comprehension. We have in the instrument of examination the actual thing to be examined: for we cannot better describe the mental life of man than as embodied in a succession of acts or states of consciousness, so continuous as to give and maintain the sense of personal identity. Whatever the forms under which we classify and describe the several mental functions, — whatever view we adopt on the much disputed question of what is innate in the mind, what derived from the senses connecting us with the external world,—equally must we come to this foundation of mental consciousness, so closely incorporate with intellectual life itself, that every other function may be held to exist only through its manifestation. *

It may seem paradoxical to speak of laws governing a part of our nature, so simple as almost to evade definition. And yet the main question before us for inquiry does so far govern all relating to individual consciousness, that its solution is connected with laws of signal interest to the philosophy of the human mind. It may be thus shortly stated: —Is our mental existence, as interpreted by consciousness, best viewed and understood as a series of acts and states, single at the same instant of time, succeeding each other with more or less rapidity of change, but in absolute and unbroken sequence? — or as a wide and mixed current, in which various sensations, thoughts, emotions, and volitions do actually coalesce and coexist as to time, and are simultaneously testified to us by this common consciousness?

It could not but happen that this question should have been often touched upon; open as it is to the cognisance of every human being; furnishing materials to the fancy of the poet; and, above all, closely connected with the

---

* The *Cogito, ergo sum*, of Descartes is only one mode of expressing this fact. The *Ichikeit* of certain German authors is an unsubstantial refinement upon the same idea; and the definition of Fichte might come more appropriately from the writings of the scholastic ages than from those of our own time. " Ursprünglich ist nur eine Substanz, *das Ich*. In dieser einen Substanz sind alle möglichen Accidenzen, also alle möglichen Realitäten gesetzt."

researches both of the metaphysician and physiologist.* The doctrine of Association of Ideas can in no wise be discussed without some reference to it, though this reference has rarely been very precise; the notion of sequence being, for the most part, lost in that of mere relation or connexion. Even more closely blended, as we have seen, is the question of Personal Identity, upon which so much learning and ingenuity have been bestowed.† Neverthe-less, this subject, as it appears to me, has not yet been so clearly defined, or explicitly treated, as its importance merits. No adequate attention has been given to the singleness or exclusiveness of particular acts of mind — or to the rapidity of their succession — or to the conditions which produce and govern their change of state — or to the influence of the will, as the most important of these conditions. Yet each one of these points involves con-clusions of great interest; and though the nature of the subject, which becomes a sort of analysis of mental exist-

---

* Whenever poetry and philosophy come into contact, as in every other case, the language of Shakespeare is always that which best describes the reality of things. He thus pictures the minutes which make up our lives : —

" Each changing place with that which goes before,
    In sequent toil all forwards do contend."

† No writer has brought to this abstruse subject more genius and learning than the late Dr. Thomas Brown. His lectures on Personal Identity, in the work published after his death, well deserve perusal; both in themselves and in their connexion with the particular subject of this chapter. Müller, in his Elements of Physiology, when treating of the Association of Ideas, has some excellent observations which bear directly on the subject before us; although not giving a systematic form to the question, and sometimes obscuring it by certain material analogies, applied to cases which do not require, and will hardly bear, such illustration.

E

ence, forbids the hope of certainty in such conclusions, yet
is the approximation sufficient to warrant full inquiry.
Whatever the power of comprehension of the mind at
each instant of time, it is clear that there is a limit to the
number of objects coexisting to the consciousness. How
near this limit approaches to unity can never, perhaps, be
proved or defined; but we may proceed far in the direction towards it, with constant reference to Time as one
of the most important elements in the question.

The first appeal to common experience here would probably not accord with that derived from closer examination. The conception conveyed under the old phrase of
Νους κυκλος is that most natural and simple. The mind in
one sense is truly a circle, comprehending not merely
things present, but the knowledge and thousand memories
of the past. It is a circle which encloses within its
boundary the faculties that have given fame to the foremost of our species — the intellect, the imagination, the
memory, the vigour of will and action, the moral feeling
of the beautiful and good. Or, to reduce the question to
particular instances, shall we doubt the comprehensive
nature of that wonderful agent, which can grasp all the
conditions of a profound mathematical problem, logically
pursue a difficult and perplexed subject of thought, resolve
by connected experiment the most abstruse questions in
physical science, or give unity and harmony to some great
work of the imagination?

With free admission of all these things, the question,
as already stated, is still open before us, and the language
of common use cannot be allowed to obscure it. In what
manner and in what degree are the mental acts, in the

cases just cited, really coincident? What is simultaneous, what belongs to simple sequence? An actual sequence, as testified and measured by time, cannot be denied. The fact belongs to common experience. May not a more minute analysis by consciousness so resolve this time into parts, and so distribute the mental phenomena along them, as to render the conception of a line more applicable than that of a circle to their manner of existence? And is this conception really at variance with the acknowledged endowments of the human mind, and those higher faculties especially which give man his supremacy among the forms of organic being on the globe?* The mind, indeed, in its entire sense, cannot be thus described. The manner of its action only is represented by a series of states, in the character and order of succession of which we may find all the elements of the highest mental power.

The simple fact of sequence being necessarily admitted, any question on this subject must have relation either to the rapidity of succession, or to the exclusiveness of the particular state of mind at each instant of time. The latter will readily be seen as the point of chief difficulty; least capable of being defined by language, and least certain in the conclusions it involves. Nevertheless much may be attained by the scrutiny of individual consciousness, directed inwards upon its own operations; the only

* Similes in matters of this kind often do more to mislead than illustrate. The subject lies too deep to be thus approached. But if any were admissible here, we might aptly, perhaps, liken the mind to a storehouse, more or less richly replenished; with many doors of ingress and egress, but the power of passage through one only at each moment of time. The metaphor might be carried further; but after all it is feeble, and furnishes no argument as to fact.

source of knowledge on this subject, as we have already seen. And here one important result will immediately occur. The closer the examination is pressed, the more will what appeared as compound resolve itself into parts— the more limited and special will be found each particular stage or state of consciousness, whether of perception, or thought, or feeling. This fact must be steadily kept in view, as of main consequence in the argument. A person, unaccustomed to such self-inquiry, may well be amazed by its results, by the incessant change of objects before his mind, the rapidity and abruptness with which they are often shifted, and the imperfect power of his will over their succession. I have known some curious cases of the wonder felt by those, who thus examine for the first time the conditions under which the whole of their lives have been unconsciously passed.

It may be alleged that in using such words as stage and state, we attempt too formally to divide and individualize what are parts of a continuous series. This may be so; but the difficulty is one of language rather than of fact. The acknowledged changes of state are in themselves acts of division; and the individuality of each, as we have just seen, is more clearly recognised as the examination becomes more minute.

But another question here occurs. How are we to define this individuality? What constitutes the single-ness of an object, as present to the mind?—an abstruse question, it must be owned, whether applied to objects of perception or thought, and hardly admitting a definite answer. Material objects, the most simple in one sense, are compound and complex in others. An idea, an image,

a memory of the mind, can scarcely be defined so as to
exclude multiplicity of parts.   Questions upon these
matters formed at once the glory and the reproach of the
scholastic ages ; but have happily been simplified or aban-
doned in the greater exactness of modern science.*   For
their bearing upon our subject it will be enough to state
generally that a physical compound may be in effect a
unit to the sense, but that no analysis of ours can reach
the exact determination of this ; or show with certainty
what objects are really individual to the perception, what
affect the mind by successive acts of sense.   When we
say that the colours and form of a simple object are perceived separately and successively, we denote at once the
minuteness of this analysis, and the impossibility of pursuing it through its ultimate stages.

Connected with this is another preliminary very
essential to the success of these investigations.   We must
thoroughly imbue ourselves with its relation to the element of time.   All phrases regarding this relation, which
custom, carelessness, or exaggeration have brought into our
language, become causes of confusion here ; nor do hours
or minutes afford any just or practical aid to our research.
We have to consider time, not as measured by the mechanism of instruments, but as an element almost infinitely
divisible, through which our existence is carried forwards
in a continuous, but ever-changing line.   Physical science

---

* We should run into the old dispute of the Nominalists and
Realists were we to pursue this particular point further.   It is one of
the many cases where words gradually usurp the place of ideas ; and
" like the Tartar's bow, shoot back upon the understanding of the
wisest."

based on mathematics, places before us many determinate divisions of time, far transcending all human conception in their minuteness. Mental science, from its nature, affords no exact measure of this kind. But though we cannot reduce to numbers, or even to any certain comparison with each other, the successive states which constitute the identity of life, we are called upon to admit a possible and frequent rapidity of change which consciousness itself can hardly follow, and with which articulate speech is wholly unable to keep pace.

I dwell upon this point, because here we are to look for the solution of those innumerable cases where it seems impossible to dissever our existence into single acts or stages of consciousness, —moments in which sensations, thoughts, memories, and emotions, crowd so together, and seem so inextricably blended, as to repel every idea of separation. Yet a reasonable inference from the analysis we are able to effect, justifies the belief that it might be carried much further, even into those evanescent portions of time, which escape our consciousness in their passage : and such inference will probably derive confirmation from the illustrations to which we are about to proceed.

These illustrations of the general views already given may best include a few pointed examples from each class of mental phenomena ; which I make of familiar kind, that they may more readily be tested by experience, and become the means of suggesting other instances. The perception by the mind of sensations from without is the topic which fitly comes first in order.

At the close of the last chapter I have adverted to the remarkable facts which designate this part of our nature

— to the individuality of successive perceptions — to the
rapid change and exclusion of one sensation by another,
the external causes remaining unaltered — to the complete
exclusion of all outward sensations during states of reflection or reverie — and to the power the mind has of selecting and arranging objects of immediate sensation.   A few
examples, illustrating these facts, will suggest innumerable
cases of similar kind.   Place yourself in the crowded
street of a city, a thousand objects of vision before the
eye — sounds hardly less various coming upon the ear —
odours also constantly changing — contact or collision at
every moment with some external object.   Amidst this
multitude of physical objects of sensation, and with all
the organs of sense seemingly open, one alone (whether in
itself simple or compound does not affect the question)
will be found at each moment distinctly present to the
mind.   It combines them only by giving close and rapid
sequence to the acts of attention.   Let the trial be made
to attend at once to the figures of two persons within the
same scope of vision ; or to listen at the same moment to
two distinct sounds ; or to blend objects of sight with those
of hearing in the same act of attention.   The impossibility
will instantly be felt, and the passage of the mind from
one act to another very often recognised.   Or, under the
same circumstances, let the mind pass suddenly, by will or
accident, into a train of inward thought, whatever the
subject ; and all the external objects thus crowded around
you utterly disappear, though the physical agents producing, and the organs receiving sensations, remain precisely as before.   Every sense sleeps, while the mind is

thus awake and active within itself. A man so occupied may be alone in a multitude.

The terms of absence of mind, abstraction, and reverie, describe analogous conditions more remarkable in character; and cases are related which might seem incredible in the separation thus made for a time between active mental existence and the material world without. Yet these instances are well authenticated, and differ but in degree from those more familiar to us. Their deep interest will readily be felt in the inferences they afford as to the various relations of our mental and corporeal nature.

In the more common examples just cited, the rapidity of change in the objects of mental perception, gives a false notion of unity of impression; which error is strengthened by the language in common use. Writing at this moment among the Eastern Pyrenees, I have before me a noble landscape of mountains, forests, river, and ruined castle, which I seek to fix firmly in my memory. In common understanding, this would be considered a single act of attention. But even did the laws of vision render it possible, it is certain that I cannot by any effort seize the totality of what is before me. I need to individualise the prominent features by rapid, but separate acts of attention, before any definite picture can be fixed upon the mind. Even the form and colouring of the objects require to be detached by perception, inseparable as they may seem to be in nature. And as the parts are thus fractionally appropriated by sense, so are they afterwards reproduced by memory, which can in no other way restore and combine the images deposited for its use.

Again, we may be in the midst of a multitude of sounds,

and one only be perceived by the sense — this, also, it may happen, instantaneously displaced by another, though the undulations which conveyed the original sensation are transmitted as before.   Or, again, if the consciousness be occupied for the time, either by some object of vision or by internal thoughts or emotions, all sounds whatsoever are lost to the ear, as if their physical causes had no existence without us.   A full orchestra may be executing a chorus of Handel while the mind is wholly absent from any consciousness of it.   The loudest roar of cannon may be annihilated at moments, to the officer who is intently engaged in manœuvring his regiment, or his ship, in the hour of battle.

The other senses furnish similar, though less striking, illustrations.   The sensations derived from our own bodily organisation are, however, well worthy of note, as cogent instances in point.   The occurrence of some new and strong sensation of this kind, is familiarly known to supersede others previously felt.   A more acute pain will frequently obliterate another before existing, though the causes of the latter are still actively present.*   Or, when suffering under severe bodily pain, if the mind be suddenly drawn away to some train of thought or moral feeling, the physical sensations will often totally cease;

---

* A curious example of this is the almost instinctive manner in which we often inflict a momentary pain, or strong sensation, upon ourselves, by pinching or otherwise, to counteract, as it were, by this voluntary infliction, the first access of pain which we know will ensue upon a blow or injury received. I recollect cases where patients have combed the head, even so as to draw blood, to obviate some distressing sensation elsewhere.

renewed only when the objects and direction of consciousness are again changed. I need not dwell, however, on
these illustrations, interesting though they are, as they
form the especial subject of the preceding chapter.

Passing now from the sensitive to the more purely
intellectual functions, the same limitation will be equally
found to exist. The mind works in a succession of acts
or states. Two thoughts, or acts of memory, however
closely related to one another, cannot be presumed to
exist at the same instant — each has its individuality in
time. Association of ideas, as already remarked, always
involves succession; nor can we otherwise understand or
define it. Experiment, in this case, might seem easy,
where the facts in a general sense are familiar to every one.
But it is made difficult by the circumstance that time is
in progress during the trial to which we put the consciousness; and that this very direction of consciousness is, in
fact, a third state in which we place the mind for the
purpose of examination. Swiftness of succession naturally
suggests a unity of time and state, which has no real
existence. In a rapid process of reasoning—in the simple
syllogism for example — we seem to have present at once
to the mind what are, in reality, steps and stages gone
through to the conclusion. Or, again, in an impassioned
speech, the warmth of eloquence and argument may give the
aspect of concentration and singleness to that which is, in
reality, the succession, incalculably rapid, of separate intellectual acts.

A strict scrutiny of consciousness will afford proof of all
this; as of the other innumerable conditions of thought,
reasoning, memory, and association, which make up the

wonderful whole of our intellectual being. Nor is there anything to degrade the mind of man in thus regarding its manner of operation. The fact of succession of ideas is indisputable. In estimating this succession by intervals of time too short to be appreciable, we bring in no new principle, but simply better define what is rarely recognised in its full import and extent.

A reasonable question may arise here as to certain cases, where two intellectual processes, perfectly distinct in themselves, appear to be absolutely simultaneous in progress; as where a person performing a difficult piece of music, converses freely at the same time on some subject wholly alien to this occupation. The explanation in this case (and applying to many others also) is, that it can only occur where the performer is so far familiar with his instrument and music, that the act becomes, in some sort, an automatic one, like the associated movements of muscles in walking, speaking, writing, &c. The element of time, too, is doubtless concerned in the explanation. The consciousness passes with inappreciable rapidity from one subject to the other, giving the effect of being simultaneous to what is in reality a succession of states. In many instances this is obvious; and such cases illustrate others, where no observation can follow the rapidity of the change.

What has been already stated applies no less to thought associated with emotion. Be the condition that of pleasure or pain, equally is it subject to the same succession, change, and exclusion. The phrases of common use in regard to human passions may colour this differently; but language is here again a false interpreter. Certain it is that the most acute feelings, the causes still subsisting, may utterly quit the mind at moments when other objects force themselves upon it; recurring afterwards with the same intensity as before. Few but have had experience of the fact, and known the pain of such sudden recurrence after the interval interposed. In the same way we explain the anomaly that pleasures or pains may be multiplied upon one another, yet produce little further effect on the feelings. The mind cannot maintain two impressions simultaneously; and, though the succession in such case may be uniformly pleasurable or painful, still it is sequence, and not coalescence of effects. Further than this, experience tells us that a new and stronger emotion will often totally obliterate a weaker one existing before; all the facts thus concurring to illustrate the one general law.

We may, perhaps, now consider it sufficiently proved, that the consciousness, which gives identity to our mental existence, consists in a series of states incessantly pressing upon one another—from causes, and under conditions, which are in part external to ourselves, in part depending on the operations of the mind itself; but all so far subordinate to time, that the further we analyse them the more do we abridge their probable duration, and reduce them to a more single and exclusive form. Our view, however, is not complete without a more especial consideration of the power the mind possesses of determining and controuling this succession; a power very various in degree, but which, in its full possession, and in due exercise, involves all the highest intellectual attainments of which man is capable. Here it is that we come in close connexion with the doctrine of Association of Ideas; a phrase sanctioned to us by the use of our most eminent philosophers, and indicating a principle which governs all the phenomena of mind. Sequence, however, as before remarked, is an indispensable part of this mental operation — the only manner in which ideas can be associated together. *   The intellectual character of any mental process depends on the manner of succession, and especially on the action of the will in determining the result.

What power, then, has the mind, by volition, in regulating the succession of its states, whether those belonging to sensations from without, or to thoughts and memory within ?   It is obvious to consciousness that it is a *limited faculty ;* corresponding in this with that wonderful combination of voluntary and involuntary acts which pervades, or, rather, constitutes, every part of our existence.   It is further certain that it differs much in different individuals ; that it varies in the same individual at different times ; that it may be enlarged by effort and cultivation ; that it is very prone to fall under the dominion of habit.   All these conditions are familiar to our experience ; but it is needful to bring them together to show their relation to each other, and to the more general laws of our nature.

In examining how far the will can govern the succession of states, which we have seen to be thus unceasing in change, it may be well to take separately the two great functions of perception and thought — and with respect to

* There are many cases where the phrase of *Succession of ideas* might advantageously be substituted for *Association ;* as expressing what is most essential in the operation, and simplifying thereby many things which are obscure without the admission of the element of time.

the first, some curious phenomena of sensation present
themselves, which do not appear to have been sufficiently
noticed, though open to observation at every moment of
life.   A certain class of these phenomena form the subject
of the preceding chapter; those, to wit, which depend on
the direction of the consciousness, by voluntary effort, to
different parts of the body.   But there are others, connected with our perceptions of the outer world, where
the exercise of the will upon objects of sensation involves
many singular results, well deserving of study.

These may be expressed generally, as the power of the
mind, by will, to select and arrange the objects of its
present perception.   They have been alluded to in several
of the examples already given; though not explicitly as the
results of volition, in which light we have now to consider
them.   Place a complex group of objects before the field
of vision; and by the will, directing the attention, we can
separate one portion of this group from the rest, so as to
make it exclusively, for a time, the subject of perception.
An assemblage of forms and shades, which would be
equally reflected by a mirror, and leave a complete delineation on a photographic surface, may afford to the mind
and memory but the single object, or grouping of objects,
to which the attention has been directed.   In like manner
we can, by volition, fix the consciousness upon one voice
amidst many, in a crowded and noisy conversation; or
upon one instrument or part in a numerous concert of
music; and pursue them continuously for a time to the exclusion of others.   When many objects are pressing at
once on the sense of touch, the mind can readily individualise one, so as to make it the sole subject of present

sensation. In these and similar cases, however, there are physical limits to the exercise of this faculty. It is needful that the objects of sense, simultaneously present, be not too numerous or intricate, otherwise the power of selection by voluntary attention becomes embarrassed or lost. And further, if the effort of attention be too long protracted, fatigue and confusion are certain to ensue; and the voluntary power, as in every other case of its exercise, gradually gives place to those automatic and involuntary actions which are continually pressing upon every part of our existence.

I know no simpler or more striking illustration of these curious phenomena than an experiment I have often made, and which any one may readily repeat and vary for himself. Let the eye be thrown upon a paper of a certain definite pattern covering the walls of a room, or on a carpet regularly figured. Though the pattern is one and the same as received on the retina (the direction of the axis of vision remaining unaltered), yet by special and separate acts of voluntary attention to different portions of it, two or three distinct patterns may often be successively obtained from the single and unchanged surface — each producing for the time a separate impression on the mind. All the subordinate details of this experiment are interesting and instructive in proportion to their simplicity. First, a considerable and often difficult effort is required for making the translation from one pattern to another. More or less time is always needed for this, and sometimes the effort fails altogether. Certain patterns favour the effort much more than others. A few well-marked opposite lines of direction and contrasted colours in the objects

delineated, would seem the conditions giving most facility
to the act; but if the configuration before the eye be
too complex and crowded, the change in the perception
cannot readily be produced. Further; there is usually
some difficulty in retaining any one of these impressions
fixedly before the mind, so that it does not blend with, or
pass into, the others; and the effort to this effect often
becomes a curious conflict between the will and the various
images pressing upon the sense.

Or, again, as regards the sense of hearing. A monoto-
nous sound may, by an endeavour of will, — not, however,
without a certain laborious effort, — be occasionally made
to take a rhythmical form, or even to combine itself into
the notes of some well-known musical air. This instance,
however, is more ambiguous than the former ; and seemingly blends itself with that other faculty by which the
mind creates or revives within itself images, or repetitions
of impressions, originally derived from the senses — selecting and grouping them together, though more obscurely
than the perceptions directly obtained from without.

The facts just stated I obtain from my own experience.
But experiments of this kind, which may be endlessly
varied, should be made on themselves by all who desire
knowledge on this curious subject. It will probably be
found that there is great diversity in different persons as
respects the faculty of thus selecting and grouping objects
of sensation; a diversity, as already remarked, common to
every exercise of the will. Such differences are interesting matters of study ; though less important than those to
which we have now to advert, before closing the subject of
this chapter.

The power which the mind can exercise by volition over
the succession of its thoughts, independently of all action
from without, is indeed a point of deep interest to the
intellectual history of man.   The power manifestly exists,
however we may name or define it.   But as manifestly is
it limited and controlled in its exercise by conditions
inherent in our nature; and mainly, it may be said, by
connexion with our bodily organisation; with the senses;
and with those functions of organic or automatic life which
are made the instruments of our being, and from which the
mind can never long or completely detach itself.   The intervention of impressions on the organs of sense; bodily
disorder or disease; and the fatigue of the mind itself,
are all concerned in this unceasing conflict between the
will and the material conditions which surround it.   These
causes, again, operate in very different degree in different
cases; producing a great disparity in the exercise of the
power, independently of that original and innate diversity
which may be presumed with certainty to exist, though
we cannot directly prove it.

Among the endless illustrations which suggest themselves here, we may find an apposite one in the simple act
of recollection; where the mind puts itself into a train of
consecutive thoughts to obtain hold of some object which
is likely to fall into the succession.   The singular manner
in which, by retrograde acts, we can retrace a long series
of associations — connected often by the slightest links —
is familiar to every one.   The object sought for is frequently thus found.   But often, also, the effort is frustrated
by disturbance from external impressions, or by internal

F

conditions of body, or by the weariness and confusion
which come upon the mind from the trial unavailingly prolonged. All this is familiarly known; and we further know
that in such cases it is best to suspend all attempt for a
while, and to take the chance of recollection through a
new series when the hindrance is removed; or to trust to
that strange and inexplicable casualty which often brings
the object upon the memory when least sought for or
expected. I prefer this example to illustrate the conflict-
ing actions of the will with the more automatic machinery
which surrounds it; for the sake, at the same time, of
assigning their proper place to the great functions of
memory and recollection among the other phenomena
before us. The mental acts depending on these occupy a
large part of human life; having relation not alone to the
past or present time, but to what lies in the future. And
however variously we may name or define these acts, they
have this common association, in their continuous sequence,
which connects them all with the individuality of our
being.

The disparity in different individuals, already mentioned,
as to the power of directing and controlling the trains of
thought, is best illustrated by instances where this power
is deficient in degree. Examples to this effect are common
in the ordinary intercourse of life. We every day meet
men whose conversation is made up of rambling incongruities; who can hold to no subject consecutively; and
who seem, and actually are, incapable of regulating the
series and association of their ideas. Such minds are a
curious subject of study; and often yield more to exami-

nation than those higher intellects which have gained, either from nature or exercise, the dominion wanting to the former. An argument with persons thus deficient,—fruitless, probably, in every other respect, — becomes a sort of analysis, by which we can discover the sudden and strange aberrations of thought, the faulty associations, and the disturbances from external impressions, which, unconsciously to themselves, perplex their whole intellectual existence. For explanation of all this we must of necessity look to the original constitution of mind, however this be defined or understood. And in the same cause we shall see why it is impossible ever completely to remedy the defect we have described.

This brings us to the only remaining question in our argument — one which may be discussed in a few words. Can this voluntary power over the course and succession of mental states —thus varying in different individuals, and limited in all, —be exercised and cultivated in such way as to enlarge its scope, and give it greater energy to resist the causes which control it? Experience answers at once, and unequivocally, that it may be so. The faculty in question is given us not merely to use, but to educate and exalt. It is eminently capable of cultivation by steady intention of mind and habitual exercise; and, rightly thus exercised, it becomes one of the highest perfections of our moral and intellectual being. By no quality is one man better distinguished from another than by the mastery acquired over the subject and course of his thoughts — by the power of discarding what is desultory, frivolous, or degrading; and of adhering singly and

steadily to those objects which enlarge and invigorate the
mind in their pursuit.*

In closing this chapter I would repeat once more that it
is no new theory of mind we have been discussing here;
but simply the *manner and course of action,* in reference to
each other and to the external world, of those various
faculties with which we are endowed. All the facts
brought forward are more or less familiar to common
observation. My object has been solely that of supplying
what I think to have been hitherto a deficiency in the
study of these phenomena, by reducing them to more distinct order, and referring them to a common principle, viz.
that of succession in time. I feel assured, on my own
experience, that the method of considering the subject
which this principle involves is one greatly tending to
give facility to research, and exactitude and truth to our
conclusions in every part of mental physiology.

---

* Magni est ingenii revocare mentem a sensibus, et cogitationem a
consuetudine revocare."—*Cicero. Tuscul. Quæst.*

CHAP. IV.

ON TIME, AS AN ELEMENT IN MENTAL FUNCTIONS.

In the last chapter I have followed through all its details that view of the mental functions which regards them as operating in series, or succession of states, from the beginning to the end of life — each single object or act of consciousness excluding for the moment all others, even of those which come most closely in precedence or sequence to it. The course of the argument has shown how closely this great element of time is concerned in every part of it; the succession of events in definite parts of time being indisputable, whatever the causes which link these events together in order and association. Yet, while common language and feeling recognise the fact at every moment, it has been too little regarded by physiologists and philosophers; seeing how fertile the topic is in curious results, and how important to a right view of the mental functions both in health and disease.

What I have still to say on the subject might have been included in this previous discussion of it, but at the expense of interfering more or less with the singleness of the argument. For of these remaining points, some relate to the changes made in the mental acts by disease — others, again, involve the consideration of time, as connected with mental operations, in a sense more general and abstract than was needful for the subject already discussed. While

thus detaching these topics, however, I must speak of
them as so closely connected with what has gone before,
that their separation can only be justified by the greater
convenience of the arrangement.

In many cases of affection of the sensorium—as in the
progress of recovering from apoplectic seizure, or generally in cases of partial coma,—a certain and often considerable time may be observed to elapse between a question
asked of the patient and his reply. And this seemingly
without any uncertainty as to the answer to be given, or
any apparent fault in the act of articulation, except slowness and greater effort—but, rather, as if the mind
received the perception more tardily than is usual or
natural—or more slowly put itself into action through
the external organs in reply. Occasionally, though aware
of the fact from former experience, I have been led by the
length of the interval to ask another question before the
first was answered; this answer following afterwards, as if
no such second question had intervened. Several cases
I have noted where a full minute has passed before the
organs were put into motion for articulate reply.

The fact here stated will be familiar to all who are
observant of cases of this kind, and it suggests at once
the most important of the questions before us. Is there
not, in reality, a material variation in the time in which
the same mental functions are performed by different individuals, or by the same individual at different times;
depending on original organisation, varying conditions of
the sensorium, or other causes of which we can give no
account? And this, not merely in complex acts of asso-

ciation, or continuous trains of thought (where the notion
of such difference is sanctioned by phrases of common use,
and can hardly be rejected), but also in the rapidity with
which perceptions are received from the senses, and volitions carried into effect on their appropriate organs — or,
in other words, both in acts purely mental and in those
functions by which the mind is associated with material
phenomena?

While finding cause to infer this fact from comparison
of individuals, the inference becomes still more distinct
and remarkable-from comparison of states in the same
person; and from that examination of consciousness which
every one may make for himself. It will be felt that
there are moments when the perceptions and thoughts are
not only more vivid, but seem to pass more rapidly and
urgently through the mind, than at other times — and the
same is felt with respect to acts of the voluntary power.*
It is possible, indeed, that these two conditions of time and
intensity are so far connected together, that one may
become a sort of measure of the other; but this would
carry the discussion into points too subtle and metaphysical
for our present purpose. The consideration of time in its
application to mental phenomena, — though appearing
simple at first view, from their being all included under it,
— does in truth involve much of abstruse inquiry; well

---

* Locke intimates something to this effect when saying, "There
is a kind of restiveness in almost every one's mind. Sometimes, without perceiving the cause, it will boggle and stand still, and one cannot
get it a step forward ; and at another time it will press forward, and
there is no holding it in."—We read in Lord Bacon of "that youth
of thought, when imaginations stream into the mind better, and, as it
were, more divinely."

fitted, however, to repay those who love the indulgence of such speculations.

It may be right to notice here the question, lately raised or revived, as to the velocity of nervous action in its simplest physical sense; and the possible diversity of this in different persons, and even in different nerves of the same individual. An apparent sanction has been given to the reality of such differences, by the singular facts which M. Nicolai, of the Manheim Observatory, records respecting the variation of time in the observation of a simple and single astronomical fact (the transit of a star across the micrometer thread of a fixed telescope), as noted by different observers on the same spot. The inequality, however, indicated by these observations, is far too great to admit of its being supposed dependent on unequal rate of transmission by the nerves of vision and hearing:— and Müller's solution is probably correct, which supposes the perceptions from the eye and ear in this case to be distinct and successive states of mind, with varying intervals between them in different individuals; a solution which accords with the view just given, and with all that we know of these mental phenomena.*

Pursuing our subject now into further details, we find many facts to illustrate it in the state of health — as many (and more striking, from being less familiar,) under morbid conditions of the body. In extreme old age, which variously expresses, through the effects of gradual change, the more sudden but transient anticipations of disease, there appears to exist not merely an impairment of the

* See Dr. Baly's valuable translation of Müller's Handbuch der Physiologie, p. 680.

powers of perception and volition, but also of those actions, whatever their nature, upon which association and sugges- tion depend.   The train of thought may be just in its order and conclusions, but it is more slowly pursued.   A longer time, in the strict meaning of the phrase, is required for those connexions, and changes by succession, which occur in every such continuous action of mind.   Here, too, as in disease, there is more of toil and difficulty in all intellectual operations,—from the simple act of attention to the more complex ones of association and thought.   The mind speedily becomes fatigued, the chain is broken, and confusion ensues.   Observation shows these occurrences, in every shade and degree, in the medical cases which come before us; and they often afford the most curious and unexpected analysis of mental conditions, which in their more perfect and healthy state seem to be indissolubly united.

It has been supposed by some that the state of dreaming involves a more rapid course of ideas through the mind;— a vague notion, however, as every thing that relates to the εθνος ονειρων seems destined to be; and incapable of any thing like proof.   All we can affirm here is, that the tran- sitions are more frequent and abrupt than in the waking state, when the regulation of the will is present; and that, as respects rapidity in the succession of thoughts, it is probably as various during sleep as at other times.   The evidence of such variation, while we are awake, is much more decisive.   We derive it from consciousness in our- selves, and observation of the minds of others; and we are frequently able to apply a certain measure to these mental changes by their relation to things without.

One particular topic, rising out of this general view of measure by time, and adverted to in the last chapter, has not been so much considered, as its interesting nature, and relation to all the mental functions, might have rendered likely. This is, the variation in the faculty of the mind of holding one single image, or thought, continuously before it, as the subject of consciousness or contemplation. The limit to this faculty in all men is certain, and in most cases narrower than is generally supposed. The persistent retention of the same idea manifestly exhausts the mind, and the effort persevered in beyond a given time will often entirely obliterate it. But nevertheless the power as to time is very various in different individuals; is susceptible of cultivation; and, if cultivated, with care not to produce exhaustion in the discipline, becomes a source of some of the highest excellences of our moral and intellectual nature. It stands contrasted with that desultory and powerless state of mind which is unable to regulate its own workings, or to retain the thought fixedly on points most essential to its object.

In all these instances we have the element of time entering, more or less directly, into our view of the mental functions engaged. Active disease here, as in so many other cases, by disturbing the relation of these different functions,—exalting some and depressing others,—affords results more strongly marked than we can obtain in the state of health; and frequent examples, involving the same notion of time, will occur to all who are sedulous in watching these changes. I have seen within the last few hours a case of typhus mitior, in which the tendency had just come on to confusion and slight delirious rambling;

where, though each question I put was rightly answered in the end, it seemed as if the mind had a long process to go through in attaining this. A case lately occurred to me, in a patient about sixty; where, without any actual paralysis, there had come on great enfeeblement of the sensorial functions, disordered perceptions, confusion of thoughts, and impaired voluntary power; but the condition as to all these points, as so often happens, varying much at different times. Here the patient himself expressed strongly the consciousness of time and labour being necessary for each voluntary act. He felt, to use his own words, " as if it were necessary to think for every finger in using it." A similar description I have often obtained from paralytic patients; indicating the slow and toilsome effort of volition required to give motion to the limbs, or other organ affected by the disease.

All this is obvious indeed to common observation. Every one must have noticed the slowness, as well as difficulty, with which the tongue is put out, the eyelids raised, or words uttered by patients in a semi-comatose state. It seems as if a certain time were needed, either for concentration or transmission of nervous power, before the intended action can be begun — while so much labour is necessary in pursuing it, that I have repeatedly observed perspiration breaking out from the continued effort to raise a palsied arm; and an exhaustion to follow, such as might ensue in health upon violent muscular exercise of the whole body. How striking the contrast here to that instant and free effort, by which action is evolved, almost simultaneously to all sense with the external impression producing it, though various mental and bodily operations actually intervene.

In another case, where there had been hemiplegia of two years' standing — the memory of words, and power of articulation, being both impaired, but the intellect un-affected—the singularity occurred of the frequent omission of one or more of the first syllables, in words of any length.   On examination, aided by the patient himself, I found cause to believe that the mind here was occasionally conceiving words more rapidly than it could put the organs into motion to express them; and there existed an in-voluntary propension to remedy this difficulty by passing at once to the sounds terminating the words.   Here then, also, if rightly interpreting the circumstances, time entered as an element into the action of the mind on the bodily organs.   These paralytic disorders, indeed — varying, as they do, in origin, progress, and in the parts affected — abound in curious examples, expressing the same general fact in different ways.   I have many such in my notes or recollection ; but as they essentially resemble those just stated from recent observation, I need not detail them.

An estimate of the different duration of time required for the same operations of mind, under different conditions of the individual, would be interesting matter of inquiry ; but exactness could scarcely be looked for, where the circumstances are so complicated.   Instances like those just given, afford a sort of rude measure for one class of cases in which disease is concerned.   And these, it must be added, are the cases showing most distinctly the origin of the diversity in physical causes.   The parts ministering to the mental functions undergo change ; and those especially which, through sensation and volition, connect the mind with the material world without. The more explicit instances furnished by disease or decay, explain, by close analogy, the natural conditions of health; nor can we reasonably doubt that the varying quickness of perception, thought, and voluntary power are as much dependent on momentary changes in the brain and nerves, as are the states of sleep and waking; with which, indeed, their connexion is in every way so intimate. Under this general view there is no greater difficulty in the notion of time, than in that of intensity or vigour, as applied to describe the progress of mental operations; though perhaps less familiar to us in reasoning on the subject.

CHAP. V.

ON SLEEP.

IT concerns not less the physician than the metaphysical
inquirer, to learn all the conditions of this remarkable
function of life, and the causes by which they are modified.
Remarkable it may fitly be called; for what more singular
than that nearly a third part of existence should be passed
in a state thus far separate from the external world! — a
state in which consciousness and sense of identity are
scarcely maintained; where memory and reason are equally
disturbed; and yet, with all this, where the fancy works
variously and boldly, creating images and impressions
which are carried forwards into waking life, and blend
themselves deeply and strongly with every part of our
mental existence.* It is the familiarity with this great
function of our nature which prevents our feeling how
vast is the mystery it involves; how closely interpreting
all the phenomena of mental derangement, whencesoever
produced; and, yet further, how singularly shadowing
forth to our conception the greater and more lasting

---

* " Half our days we pass in the shadow of the earth, and the
brother of death extracteth a third part of our lives," says Sir Thomas
Browne; a writer whose genius and eloquence give him a high
place in English literature, as well as in that of the profession to
which he belonged.

changes the mind may undergo without loss of its individuality.

I am not sure that the subject, in its medical relations, has even yet received all the notice it deserves. Much knowledge, indeed, has been gained of late, by looking more closely into the physical connexions of sleep with other actions of the body; and especially with those functions of the nervous system to which it is most intimately allied. But there is still scope for a few remarks, having reference partly to the physiology of sleep, and its relations to these particular functions — partly to its connexion with the various forms and treatment of disease.

It is singular that in a state thus familiar, and filling so large a portion of the term of life, it should yet be difficult to distinguish that which is the most perfect condition of sleep — the furthest removed from the waking state. No certain proof can be had of this from our own recollections, nor from the feelings on awakening. Both depend more or less on the dream or other condition immediately antecedent, or even on the manner in which we are aroused from it. The best proofs, though still very ambiguous, are derived from the observation of those around. That may be presumed generally the soundest sleep in which there is seen to be most complete tranquillity of the bodily organs commonly dependent on the will. Sensation, the other great function of the brain involved, furnishes evidence to the same point in the varying effect of stimuli applied to the senses when thus closed. And this test might perhaps be the most certain, were it not that we have cause to believe the different senses to be unequally affected, even at the same moment of time: and that there is further ambiguity from the occasional passage of sleep into coma, through gradations which cannot be defined by any limits we are able to draw.*

Evidence by ready tests as to the soundness of sleep is often of value in practice; both in reference to the point last mentioned, and because the physician is very liable to be misled by the error of the patient himself on the subject. The best proof which the latter can give is the absence of consciousness of having dreamed. This, however, does not render it certain that dreams have not existed. The observation of others, and the recollections often suggested afterwards of dreams of which there has been no memory at the time, prove it to be wholly otherwise. The question as to this point, indeed, is one that has been much debated, and a decisive answer is very difficult. But I hold it as more probable, that no moment of sleep is without some condition of dreaming; — that is, that images are always present to the individual consciousness, and trains of thought founded thereon; however vague and unreal in themselves, and however slight, if any, the recollections they carry on to our waking existence. To believe it otherwise is to suppose two different states of sleep, more remote from each other than we can well conceive any two conditions of the same living being; — one, in which sensations, thoughts, and emotions are present in activity and unceasing change; — another, in which there is the absence or nullity of every function of

* Aristotle, towards the end of his Book, Περι Ενυπνιων, has some curious remarks on the subject, well illustrated by examples. All his writings on this, and other collateral topics, deserve much more intimate perusal than is given to them at the present time.

mind; annihilation, in fact, for the time, of all that is not merely organic life. Though we cannot disprove the latter view — and must admit the difficulty of explaining the sleep of an infant in any other sense — yet is it on the whole more reasonable to suppose that no state of sleep is utterly without dreaming; the actual diversity being testified chiefly, though very imperfectly, by the varying recollection of what has passed through the mind during the time in question.*

However this may be, it is very important, in all our reasonings, practical and theoretical, upon sleep, to keep in mind that it is not a unity of state with which we are dealing; but a series of fluctuating conditions, of which no two moments perhaps are strictly alike. It may even be affirmed, with certainty, that these variations extend from complete wakefulness to the most perfect sleep of which we have cognizance either from outward or inward signs. In the symptoms, as well as treatment, of disease, a due regard to this fact is often of material consequence. While, looking to the subject physiologically, it is absolutely essential to the truth of our conclusions; and will assist us, beyond any other mode of research, in explaining all the seeming anomalies of this great function of life.

Attaching such importance to this view, and seeing the familiarity of the phenomena on which it is founded, we

---

* This question is noticed expressly by Aristotle, Διά τινα αἰτίαν καθεύδοντες, ὅτε μὲν ὀνειρώττουσιν, ὅτε δὲ οὔ· ἢ συμβαῖνει μὲν ἀεὶ καθεύδουσιν ἐνυπνιάζειν, ἀλλ᾽ οὐ μνημονεύουσι. Περὶ Ὕπνου. Lord Brougham, in his Discourse on Natural Theology, holds an opinion the reverse of that stated above; and vindicates, with his wonted power of argument, the belief that we dream but during the time of transition into and out of sleep, when the two states are graduating into each other.

may well feel surprise that it should be so little regarded
in all common reasoning on the subject. We speak,
indeed, of light sleep, or heavy sleep, or broken sleep;
but these and other vague phrases (often, as we have seen,
erroneously applied) give little idea of that gradation of
states which connects the waking and sleeping life of man
— the extreme and opposite limits of his worldly being.
Long and familiar habit can alone explain this indifference.
In infancy, wonder, as an intellectual agent (and it has
not inaptly been called "the mother of knowledge " *), is
yet undeveloped. As life advances, the phenomena have become so habitual, that we satisfy ourselves with the vague
phrase of *natural;* and look carelessly on the wonderful
aspects of sleep, as we usually see it; or even when
under the comatose condition of disease. A child may be
rocked or sung into a slumber of hours. A man may be
speedily thrown into sleep by a certain posture of head,
by a full stomach, by a dull or difficult book, by a mono-
tonous sound, by repetition of numbers or forms of words,
by over exercise and fatigue of the senses. Dreams come
on, changing at every moment; various movements of the
voluntary organs; often articulate speech — yet all these
things pass unheeded before us. But let it happen that
similar conditions are produced by mesmeric passes or other
similar means, and the phenomena are looked upon with
astonishment and awe. The deep interest which rightly
belongs to sleep in its ordinary state, is excited for the
first time by the unwonted manner in which it is brought
on; and a great function of our nature, ever open to

---

* A fact well expressed long before by Aristotle, Διὰ γὰρ τὸ
θαυμάζειν οἱ ἄνθρωποι καὶ νῦν καὶ τὸ πρῶτον ἤρξαντο φιλοσόφειν. Metaphys.
i. 12.

rational inquiry, is thus mystified and obscured by the manipulations of art.

Recurring now to the view of sleep, as a succession of ever-varying states, common experience furnishes us with endless illustrations. Look, for example, to the passage from waking to sleeping, and see with what rapidity and facility these states often alternate with each other. It is in the act of transition that we may best authenticate our knowledge of these phenomena; and the most ordinary incidents are full of instruction, if the mind be directed to observe them. One familiar instance is that of being on horseback when much wearied from want of rest. Here, at every moment, the mind lapses into a dozing state, from which the loss of the balance of the body as frequently and suddenly arouses it. In this case, and in all of like kind, neither the sleep nor the waking consciousness is perfect; but the mind is kept close to an intermediate line, to each side of which it alternately passes. No such line, however, really exists; and it is merely a rapid shifting to and fro of conditions of imperfect sleep and imperfect waking, giving curious proof of the manner in which these states graduate into one another.*

Or take another common case of a person seeking rest on an uneasy bed, or under the influence of pain or disordered digestion. Obviously to himself, as to those around him, there is incessant alteration of state, testified by various

---

* Exact estimate of time is obviously difficult here; but I have frequently, when in a carriage, obtained proof that this alternation of the loss and recovery of waking consciousness must have occurred at least three times within a minute, by knowing the distance gone over while the observation was made.

bodily movements, by partial consciousness to external objects, by dreams broken and renewed — a strange interlacing of the two conditions, which thus divide our existence.

Watch again the loss of voluntary power in a person sinking quietly into sleep; — how gradual it is — how exact a measure of the state coming on. An object is grasped by the hand while yet awake — it is seen to be held less and less firmly, till at last all power is gone, and its falls away. The head of a person in sitting posture gradually loses the support of the muscles which sustain it upright : it droops by degrees, and in the end falls upon the chest. Here, again, we have proof of the rapidity with which the loss and recovery of voluntary power may alternate on the confines of sleep. The head falls by withdrawal of power from particular muscles. The slight shock thence ensuing partially awakens and restores this power, which again raises the head. It is well known how often this may be repeated within a short space of time, each such motion implying a definite alteration of the voluntary power.

The gradual changes which occur in the perceptions from the senses, while sleep is coming on, afford the same curious notices of the condition of the mind in its relations to the world without. The sight, the hearing, the touch, all show the progressive lessening of sensibility through every stage of change, with the same fluctuations which attend those of the voluntary power; and giving similar proof that the state of sleep is ever varying in degree as respects these several functions. We find, for example, one condition of sleep so light, that a question asked

restores consciousness enough for momentary understanding
and reply; and it is an old trick to bring sleepers into
this state, by putting the hand into cold water, or producing some other sensation, not so active as to awaken,
but sufficient to draw the mind from a more profound to a
lighter slumber. This may be often repeated, sleep still
going on; but make the sound louder and more sudden,
and complete waking at once ensues. The same with
other sensations. Let the sleeper be gently touched,
and he shows sensibility, if at all, by some slight muscular
movement. A ruder touch excites more disturbance and
motion, and probably changes the current of dreaming;
yet sleep will go on; and it often requires a rough shaking,
particularly in young persons, before full wakefulness can
be obtained. I have seen children pinched or pricked
sharply with a pin, without other effect than that of
making the slumber restless for a time. These various
cases, which depend severally on the intensity of sleep,
and on the kind and degree of the exciting causes without,
will be found to explain many of those mesmeric appearances which are offered to us under a widely different
interpretation.

It is certain that the faculties of sensibility and volition
are often unequally awakened from sleep. The case may
be stated, familiar to many, of a person sleeping in upright
posture, with the head falling over the breast; in whom
sensibility is suddenly aroused by some external impression,
but who is unable, for a certain time, to raise his head,
though the sensation produced by this delay of voluntary
action is often singularly distressing. The actions of

86 ON SLEEP.

the same interesting fact; and merit even more attention
than they have yet received, in reference to these and
other phenomena.*

The same mode of observation may be followed as to
the higher mental faculties, to which these functions
severally minister. The state of unconscious reverie (as
distinguished from that voluntary abstraction which a man
may exercise for the most exalted purposes) is one of the
first conditions which intervene in the progress we are
describing. The mind kept for some time, as often happens,
in a state intermediate between sleep and waking, is
capable of recognising those rapid and repeated changes
by which it shifts to each side of the imaginary line ; and
the moments of waking consciousness afford distinct and
curious notice of the slumbering moments which have
intervened — of those strange aberrations of thought ("the
mimicry of reason," as Dryden well calls them), in which
volition is dormant, and memory awake only to furnish
incongruous images to the dream.† The self-analysis we

---

* I have notes of several cases of disease, singularly illustrating
this disjunction of sensibility and volition. In one remarkable case of
a young lady, in whom, for many weeks together, a state of trance
lasting some hours came on at a certain time each day, the gradation
of change was strikingly marked. The voluntary power in moving,
speaking, &c. was wholly suspended, while the perception by the
senses still remained. These next disappeared, and the trance became
complete ; ending, after a time, in severe tetanic spasms, sometimes
reaching the state of opisthotonos. The exact uniformity in the series
of these morbid changes formed a striking circumstance in the case.
The first step towards amendment was by irregularity in their occurrence.

† Though poetry is not often admissible in aid of discussions of

can employ in this case better shows than any reasoning how completely these states graduate into each other, and to what extent the acts of the wakeful mind interpret those of the most perfect sleep. But the topic of dreaming, to which we here approach, is too large and curious to be submitted to this cursory survey; and, though hardly separable from any discussion of the nature and conditions of sleep, I must reserve to the next Chapter the observations I have to make on this subject.

The facts belonging to somnambulism afford the most remarkable illustration of the phenomena we have been recording. Though their rarer occurrence gives them the semblance of exceptional instances, they depend on similar causes, and express equally the relations by which different states of sleep graduate into one another; and into the functions of the waking state. The fact, that we can often succeed, by the excitement of external impressions, in altering the acts of the somnambulist without awakening him, is a striking proof of the various degrees in which the senses may be merged in the condition of sleep.

Bichat, whose observations on the subject have all his wonted originality of thought and language, more distinctly propounds this view of the great function of which we are treating. The phrase " Le sommeil général est l'ensemble des sommeils particulièrs" expresses his view of the nature and complexity of this state, as one in which each separate sense and mental faculty may be at the same moment in

this nature, I cannot forbear referring to some lines of Dante, which admirably express the transition we are describing : —

> " E tanto d' uno in altro vaneggiai,
> Che gli occhi per vaghezza ricopersi,
> E pensamenti in sogno trasmutai."

very different conditions, even so far, that some may be deemed awake, while others are wholly wrapt in sleep.* With slight qualification, particularly as to the latter point, this opinion must be admitted as best accordant with facts, and necessary indeed to the right explanation of the phenomena. It comes nearest to what may be termed a just theory of sleep; and any seeming deviation from simplicity in its first aspect is more than compensated by the facility it is found to give to all reasoning on the subject. The proofs are numerous, though instances of the kind already stated; and in all such examples, the simpler and more limited the circumstances, the clearer is the evidence they set before us.

Other facts still require to be noticed in illustration of these views. Though admitting sleep to come on by a series of gradations from the waking state, the consequence by no means follows that all those gradations must be gone through in the passage from one stage of sleep to another. The time occupied in transition is doubtless very different in different cases; and in many instances, particularly in certain nervous disorders, it would seem that the changes or alternations between two states remote from each other may take place with extreme abruptness; either in effect of external impressions, or from the sudden and inexplicable aberrations of dreams. It is highly probable, indeed, that the manner in which sleep is produced does much to determine its particular conditions at the moment, and even its course beyond. It may be brought on more or less suddenly; and more or less com-

---

* In conformity with this view, Bichat says of dreams, " Ils ne sont autre chose qu'une portion de la vie animale échappée de l'engourdissement où l'autre portion est plongée."

pletely, as respects the degree in which the mental functions are absorbed; and these diversities, equally observable in the passage again to the waking state, depend greatly in both cases on the circumstances under which the change of state begins. This result might have been in part inferred from the views already propounded; but it is confirmed to us by various evidence of facts; and is obviously very important in the explanation of appearances which have recently perplexed the minds of many candid observers.*

Sleep, then, in the most general and correct sense of the term, must be regarded not as one single state, but a succession of states in constant variation: — this variation consisting, not only in the different degrees in which the same sense or faculty is submitted to it; but also in the different proportions in which these several powers are under its influence at the same time. We thus associate together under a common principle all the phenomena, however remote and anomalous they may seem, from the bodily acts of the somnambulist; the vivid, but inconsequent, trains of thought excited by external impressions; the occasional acute exercise of the intellect; and the energy of emotion — to that profound sleep, in which no impressions are received by the senses; no volition is exercised; and no consciousness or memory is left, on waking, of the thoughts or feelings which have existed in the mind.

* The observations of Mr. Braid, more especially, have done much to establish this fact of the altered character of sleep in effect of the manner in which it is brought on; and this may be regarded as a valuable part of his researches.

Instead of regarding many of these facts as exceptions and anomalies, it is sounder in reason to adopt such definitions of sleep as may practically include them all. And this, which can be done in perfect accordance with just physiological views, has been the course and tendency of modern inquiry on the subject. The principle is one, not merely sound and sufficient in theory, but beneficial in many points of practice, by solving difficulties which often occur in the aspect of symptoms and treatment of disease.

In thus, too, following the various states and acts of sleeping, through their relation to those of waking existence, and tracing the gradations from one into the other, we obtain results of the same precise and practical kind as those derived from pursuing the natural and healthy functions of mind into the different forms of insanity and mental disorder. Each part of these topics, so considered, illustrates every other; furnishing suggestions which could not be derived from any other source.

In this manner, again, of viewing sleep—not as one, but a series of complex and ever-varying states—we find best explanations of those singular conditions of trances, mesmeric sleep, catalepsy, &c., which have served at all times to perplex the world by the strange breach they seem to make between the bodily and mental functions; by their unexpectedness in some cases; and by the peculiar agency producing them in others. The latter circumstance, especially, serves to disguise from us their real relation to other and more familiar affections of the nervous system. As respects magnetic sleep or trance, in particular, whatever its shape or degree, there is no authenticated fact making it needful to believe that any influence is received from with-

out; beyond those impressions on the senses and imaginations, which are capable in certain persons and temperaments of exciting unwonted or disordered actions throughout every part of the nervous system, and especially in the
sensorial functions. The whole scope of the question is
manifestly comprised in this single point.

There is not the slightest reason to deny that mesmeric
sleep may differ greatly in intensity, or other conditions,
from that of ordinary kind. The views already stated as
to the nature and infinite variety of this great function
make full allowance for such diversity; depending partly
on the manner in which the state is induced, partly on the
peculiar habit of the persons thus acted upon. Further it
is to be remarked, that this diversity is scarcely greater
than we find among the natural conditions of sleep; and
that the mesmeric sleep is itself exceedingly various in kind
and degree—from the vague state of reverie or half-trance,
in which impressions are still received from the senses, and
excite wandering actions of mind — to that deeper trance,
in which, as in coma and other anæsthetic states, even
violent stimuli applied to the body fail to awaken or produce any obvious effect. This is a condition evidently
remote from common sleep; yet differing, as far as we can
see, only in degree. The immediate gradations express
that general law of continuity which pervades and explains
all these phenomena.*

* Though the difference is presumably one of degree only, it leads
to some curious inquiries regarding sensation, from the seeming fact
that the sense of touch is that especially affected in these cases; and
that such experiments seemed chiefly in habits where this sense
readily acquires a morbid sensitiveness; as in females where the
hysteric temperament is strongly marked.

We must not quit this topic without noticing the striking
results of what has been termed *Hypnotism*—the sleep or
trance produced, not by mesmeric means, but by the act
of the individual himself, made to concentrate his vision
fixedly for a certain time upon some one object.   It apparently facilitates the effect if this object be of small size ;
and Mr. Braid's interesting experiments would seem to
show what may well be understood, that the posture of the
head further favours the results.   The simple fact, that the
various physical character of the object gazed upon does in
no way alter the effect, will readily be received as sufficient proof, that the trance induced arises from causes
within, and not from influences *without*, the body of the
person thus affected.

The evidence, indeed, furnished by these experiments in
relation to mesmeric sleep, is simple and convincing as
respects the main assumption, that this state is brought on
by the influence of one human body on another.   The
effects are less in degree, inasmuch as the means employed
less powerfully excite the imagination.   But they are expressly the same in kind ; and justify the conclusion, that
all these states depend on affections of the nervous system,
in persons of a certain temperament, and under certain
modes of excitement.*

All that relates to dreaming is of course subordinate to
the general idea we have taken of the nature of sleep.   I
have already explained why, in this chapter, I refrain

---

* These researches of Mr. Baird on Hypnotism well deserve careful
examination ; as do also his valuable experiments connected with
Electro-Biology ; each inquiry illustrating the other by analogous
facts and inferences.

from entering into any details on this curious topic, so perplexing to the reason, so exciting to the imagination. There is but one question to which I will allude, from its connexion with the inquiry into the physical conditions of sleep, — viz. why some dreams are well remembered, others not at all, or very imperfectly? Two causes, at least, may be conjectured here. One is, that in the former instance the sleep is really less complete in kind — that peculiar condition of brain less marked, upon which the imperfection of memory, if not also the exclusion of sensations, appears to depend. Another is, that the images and thoughts forming some dreams are actually stronger and deeper in their impression than those of others; — an expression too vague for use, were it not that we are obliged equally to apply it to that more common diversity of waking states, upon which the memory so much depends for all that regard its promptitude and completeness. The combination of these circumstances, with others perhaps less obvious, affords as much explanation as we can attain without more complete knowledge of the proximate causes of sleep. To the first probably we may look for interpretation of the old notion of the " *somnia vera* " of approaching day. The physical state of sleep is then less perfect; — trains of thought suggested, follow more nearly the course of waking associations — and the memory retains them, while earlier and more confused dreams are wholly lost to the mind.

The latter, however, though lost at the moment, leave traces which, like the memory of waking acts, are capable of being restored at a more remote time by new associations. There are few who have not occasionally felt certain vague and fleeting impressions of a past state of mind, of which the recollection cannot by any effort take a firm hold, or attach it to any distinct points of time or place; — something which does not link itself to any one part of life, yet is felt to belong to the identity of the being. These are not improbably the shades of former dreams; the consciousness, from some casual association, wandering back into that strange world of thoughts and feelings in which it has existed during some antecedent time of sleep, without memory of it at the moment, or in the interval since. A fervid fancy might seek a still higher source for this phenomenon, and poetry adopt such; but the explanation is probably that just given.*

The power often attained of wakening at a fixed hour depends obviously on that law of habit which governs so largely the course of all our functions, and particularly those of animal life. The time in these cases cannot be altered without creating by especial means a new habit. When on any single occasion the need of waking early produces the effect, it is merely because the sleep itself is disturbed by the dominant idea of this necessity; and is broken at repeated intervals, without any exact relation to the time required.

The question as to the physical causes of sleep, remote and proximate, has been so much discussed, that I advert to it only for the purpose of simplifying what we know on the subject. The great object in view is manifestly the reparation of exhausted power. This need extends, in the

---

* Bayle, speaking on this subject, says, "Des tels faits, dont l'univers est tout plein, embarrassent plus les esprits forts, qu'ils ne le témoignent."

most general sense, to life in every form; but applies
peculiarly to animal life, and bears some proportion here
to the higher organisation and faculties of the species.*
The law of intermittence, more distinct as we thus rise
in the scale of functions, depends upon, and provides for,
this necessity; showing itself most expressly in that periodical repose to the two great functions of sensibility and
volition which we name sleep; and which, so established,
links itself closely with every other part of our mental
and corporeal existence. It may be that the varying
conditions of this state, upon which I have so fully dwelt,
have some relation to the exhaustion of one sense or faculty
more than another; but the evidence on this point is too
obscure to justify any certain conclusions.

Considering the proximate cause under this general law,
it seems certain that it is to be found in some particular
state of the nervous substance, having close relation to
these functions; — a state different from that of waking
life, yet graduating into it on every side; — incapable,
perhaps, of being ever ascertained by observation, yet not
the less real as a change on this account. We have
proof, partly in the nature of the functions affected, which
depend immediately on this part of the organisation; partly
in the nature of the causes tending to produce sleep.
These are all such as have influence, more or less directly,
on the nervous system; — fatigue of body or mind — exhaustion by pain or other strong impressions previously
sustained — the absence of strong impressions on any of

---

* The hybernation of some animals appears as an exception to the
principle; this state, though recurring periodically, yet obviously
depending on other causes than the mere need of rest.

the senses — the action of various narcotics — particular
conditions of the blood, and of circulation through the
brain — certain stages of digestion — and, finally, certain
causes acting more directly on the nerves themselves.
The latter involve, as we have seen, some of the most
curious conditions of the animal economy; such as have
at all times tended to perplex the understanding, and
beget endless varieties of superstitious belief.

In looking to these various causes which act on the
sensorium to the production of sleep, we find again the
advantage gained by viewing this state as one of unceasing
change; not only in general intensity, but further, and
more remarkably, in the degree in which different functions and faculties are involved in it. This is especially
true as respects the influence of the circulation; the most
important of these causes, and that with which we have
greatest practical concern, from our power of modifying
its action. Knowing what we do of its frequent and
rapid changes in the waking state, it is easy to understand how similar inequalities may so act on the brain and
nervous system as to produce every degree of sleep, and
constant variation in the particular functions submitted
to it. Whether quality of blood, or the mechanical effects
of quantity, or rate of movement, be most concerned
(and there is reason from observation to admit all), equally
will any such inequalities tend to produce the effects
in question.

And here, too, we must seek explanation of many of the
irregularities of dreaming. It is certain that these greatly
depend (probably much more than the variations of the
waking state) on the fluctuating circulation through the

brain. We have many curious proofs how slight a difference of pressure, partial or general, on this organ, is
capable of producing the most singular effects on its
functions; and disturbing not only the perceptions of the
senses, but all the higher operations of mind. Dreams
are the most striking evidence and interpreters of this
fact. Where they have been singularly vivid and consecutive through the night, I believe it will generally be
found that there is some concomitant heaviness or oppression of head, indicating congestion or other disturbance of
the vascular system there. And that this operates mainly
as cause (though perhaps itself reciprocally acted upon)
may be inferred from the previous conditions likely to
disturb the circulation; and also from the frequent repetition of the same vividness of dreams, with intervals of
waking between.

It must be admitted, however, that the order of occurrences is not wholly known to us here. The actions and
reactions between the nervous system and that of the
circulation, are so numerous and complicated, that it is
impossible to decipher them in detail; or even, in many
cases, to indicate which is cause and which effect. This,
indeed, forms one great difficulty in our investigation
of the physical causes of sleep. There is no reason
to suppose it insuperable; though a more absolute limit
lies beyond, common to all researches of this nature, and
stopping every further progress in this direction.

In investigating the nature of sleep, we must advert to
the causes which prevent, as well as those which favour or
produce it. These of course are chiefly the converse of
the latter: but some of them deserve notice from the

H

further illustrations they afford. The peculiar influence of
certain substances, even of common articles of diet, as
coffee and green tea, may be mentioned among them.*
Though by no means invariable, and often blended with
other effects, yet is it distinct enough to furnish the same
inferences as those we derive from opium in its action
as a soporific. In both cases we have to presume a positive change of state, though doubtless of different kind
for each, throughout certain parts of the nervous system.
Any influence these agents can produce on the circulation,
is wholly inadequate to explain the results. We know
that opium, and other narcotic substances, have effects,
locally applied, on nervous sensibility, and the action of
the muscular fibre — and there can be little doubt that
when they produce sleep, it is the same singular influence,
extended more widely over this part of the organisation;
and reaching, through the cerebral part of it, the higher
faculties of our being.

The length of time during which maniacs, in restless or
violent activity, occasionally continue without sleep, is
among the facts which seem to baffle all speculation. If
venturing any hypothesis on the subject, it would be,
that in some kinds of mania there is an actual excess in
the production of that nervous power, by the exhaustion
of which under ordinary circumstances sleep is produced.

* The similarity of effects, and even of the peculiar sensations from
coffee and tea, adverted to in my Medical Notes in evidence of some
common principle, has since been illustrated by the researches of
Liebig and Pfaff, proving the existence of an organic base (*theine* or
cafeine) common to both; and singularly related to those other organic
bases, morphine, quinine, strychnia, &c., which are medicinal or
poisonous according to their manner of use.

Were this view, for which there are some plausible reasons, capable of being proved, it would explain why the intervention of such state (designed to give time for reparation) should be so little needed in these cases. And, even without explanation of this curious anomaly, we may receive the fact as illustrating by analogy various minor cases, where we observe diminution of sleep for considerable periods, without any proportionate waste of power. There are seemingly differences in the capacity of the sensorium at different times for the performance of its functions; similar action being attended with greater and more speedy exhaustion at one time than another. This is a fact familiar to the consciousness of every one; and which must be referred to physical variations (appreciable only by their effects) in the state of the nervous power ministering to these actions.

It is a point worthy of note, though familiar, that whereas moderate mental occupation and excitement tend to produce sleep, excess in degree or duration of this state has the effect of preventing it. And this is true, not only as to strong emotions of mind, the influence of which is at times painfully proved to every one; but even as to simple intellectual exertion, where the efforts are excessive, and too long protracted. Many remarkable instances have occurred to me in practice of habitual loss of sleep from this cause. Such effect is never to be neglected; as it is a token of what may become danger in various ways. The practical admonitions of the physician are as necessary here, as in the treatment of fever or inflammatory disease — the brain invariably suffering in the end, and in degree at all times, from exertions which produce this

H 2

result. The slighter inroads of the habit can only be detected by the patient himself; but he must be led to a right estimation of their consequences.

The influence of the previous state of mind in procuring or preventing sleep is curious in every way. Minute observation here offers many seeming incongruities, which cannot be explained without knowing better than we do its physical causes, and their relation to the sensorial functions. What seems most needful for attaining it is the disengagement of the mind from any strong emotion, or urgent train of thought. Great anxiety to bring on sleep implies these very conditions, and is therefore more or less preventive of it. The various artifices of thought and memory used for the purpose often fail from this cause. When they succeed, it depends either on the ex-haustion becoming more complete, or on the mind being rapidly carried from one object to another; — a desultory state of this kind, without emotion, being apparently the condition most favourable to the effect desired.

A great source of inequality and disturbance in sleep is doubtless to be found in the state of the viscera; and especially of those by which digestion is performed. This process, going on during sleep, carries the ingesta through successive stages of change, and through different parts of the alimentary canal; every such change, even under the healthiest action, altering in some way the state of the body, and the impression upon the sensorium; — indirectly, through the circulation — or directly, by excitement to different parts of the nervous system — or mechanically, by hindrance to the flow of blood in the great vessels, from pressure upon them in the epigastrium.

Out of this general view many particular questions arise. Such are those which regard the cause of the sleepiness directly following a full or ill-digested meal; or of the disturbance to sound sleep which often occurs in the middle of the night, six or seven hours after dinner, and is obviously connected with some part of the process of digestion. The first effect depends probably on the loaded stomach itself; and is testified by that laborious and unrefreshing sleep familiar to most persons at one period or another. The latter effect may depend on the colon becoming loaded about this time with what is received from the small intestines; performing its functions with difficulty; and from the recumbent posture creating disturbance by pressure on the great vessels and other surrounding parts. All such effects of digestion upon sleep are strikingly attested by its influence on dreaming; and they are of course greatly varied in kind, and augmented in degree, from any actual disease of the organs concerned. Restless nights form one in the long catalogue of distresses of the dyspeptic patient, and aggravate greatly the evils out of which they arise. Medicine in its dietetic part may do much here; nor is the physician to disregard any means as trifling which can minister to so great a good.

Whatever of wholesome change in diet may have been made in this country of late years, there is cause to think that we deal injuriously with the night by bringing the time of dinner so closely upon it. The interval of four or five hours between the heaviest meal of the day, and the time of going to bed, is by no means that most favourable to sound rest. The early stage of digestion is passed

over, during which there is natural tendency to repose;
and we seek it at a time when the system, as respects the
influence of food, is taking up again a more active state;
and when exercise, rather than the recumbent posture, is
expedient in forwarding healthily the latter stages of this
process.   The old method of supper at bed-time, in sequel
to dinner in the middle of the day, was probably better in
regard to the completeness of rest at night; and the
habit of good sleep may often be retrieved by adopting a
plan of this kind, when every anodyne has failed of effect.
With all the facility the human body has of adapting
itself to change of circumstances, there are cases where
this can never wholly be done.   And the connexion of
digestion with sleep is so important and unceasing, that
we have every cause to infer some relation as to time
between the two functions, better fitted than any other
to fulfil healthily the purposes of both.   This it is the
business of the physician to ascertain; and though he
cannot change the course of worldly habit in these matters,
the knowledge so gained may at least become an important aid in the treatment of disease.

The close dependence of sleep on the state of the alimentary canal makes it probable that evil is often incurred
by giving purgatives habitually at bed-time.   The custom
is a common one; and not least so in dyspeptic cases.
Yet here especially every thing ought to be avoided which
by irritation can disturb the soundness of rest; — a consequence often inevitable of the action on the membranes
which aperient medicines produce. Benefit may frequently
be gained in such cases, by changing the time of using
these remedies, where they cannot be dispensed with
altogether.

The relation of sleep to perspiration is a point of importance in the animal economy. It seems certain that this secretion or transudation, however it be termed, is augmented in a certain degree by sleep, independently of the influence of external causes.* The fact is connected with and illustrates certain of the phenomena of fever; and is capable in various ways of practical application. There is reason to believe that this is the true cause of perspiration in very many cases, where medicines given to procure it receive credit for the effect.

The influence of different diseases upon sleep, as well as the reciprocal effects of disturbance in this function, form a curious subject of inquiry; but so extensive and complex, that it can scarcely be pursued on any general principle. An important topic here is the relation of sleep to disorders of the brain; with some of which it has close kindred both in the functions affected, and in the apparent manner in which this takes place. There are many instances in which it would be difficult to recognise any other distinction than that of duration; though, from the difference of cause which this presumes, we may infer that

---

* The multiplied observations of Sanctorius and Keill on this subject are confirmed by the more recent inquiries of Dr. Edwards. The labours of Sanctorius in these parts of physiology are scarcely enough regarded at the present time. Two or three particular results are quoted and requoted from him; without due notice of the vast mass of observations he collected; with singular diligence and fidelity, and often by very curious and instructive means of research. The modern method (for such it may be termed) of applying averages to results of this kind, is indispensable, where the conditions are so numerous and so complicated with each other.

other variations really exist. It is certain that the states
of sleep and coma frequently graduate into each other,
in such way as to show that the proximate physical conditions are nearly the same in both. Either name may
be given to the state produced by moderate pressure on
the brain, when a portion of the cranium is removed. In
a remarkable example of this kind, which I saw in one
of the English military hospitals at Santarem, when tra-
velling in Portugal in 1812, there was cause from observation to infer, that the patient went through every grade
between these conditions, in proportion to the degree of
pressure applied. And instances are probably common to
the same effect, though always liable to some doubt in
their interpretation.*

The judgment of the physician is often embarrassed in
these cases; and practical injury may be the consequence
of error. It is an observation of Dr. Wilson Philip, that
no sleep is healthy but that from which we are easily
aroused. And though the remark requires to be qualified
by the consideration that sleep may be too light in kind
to fulfil its purposes in the animal economy, it justly
points out the opposite excess, and a state too closely
verging on the conditions of brain which endanger apo-
plexy. Changes of circulation in the head, however produced, are doubtless concerned in all these variations.
The aid often obtained in bringing on sleep by placing the
head low, and the difficulty of sleeping in an upright

---

* The experiments of Flourens, who produced a state resembling
sleep by removing portions of the cerebrum, must be admitted
under the same suspicion which attaches to almost all observations
thus made.

posture, are familiar proofs how much the state of the
brain in sleep is determined by the general manner of circulation through it, independently of all partial inequalities.
One degree of pressure seems essential to perfect and
uniform sleep; while a greater degree, without other
alteration of state, assumes more or less the character of
disease. The best inferences, in relation to practice, are
generally to be derived from notice of other symptoms;
particularly from the degree of sensibility present, from
the state of respiration, and from the manner of action of
the heart.

I have already alluded to the probable effect of the
quality, as well as quantity and distribution, of the blood
upon the various states of sleep; and may notice it again
as one of the modes in which this natural function is
affected by the presence and fluctuations of disease. There
is reason to suppose that such effects chiefly depend on
the proportion of venous blood present in the cerebral
circulation, either from congestion in the great veins, or
from imperfect arterialization in the lungs. But there are
other changes less easily recognised than these — depending on the casual presence of foreign matters in the blood,
or more frequently on the imperfect separation of those
ingredients which it is the business of the excreting organs
to remove — the existence of which diffuses disorder
throughout the system; affecting the sleep frequently in
such way as to give it the characters of a morbid state,
sometimes verging on dangerous disease.

Through this latter view more especially we are enabled
to interpret the remarkable relation between the functions
of the kidneys and the state of sleep; a subject not suffi-

ciently regarded by physicians, though attested by constant and familiar observations, and illustrated by those more serious cases, where renal disease produces disorders of the brain; of which sleep, heavier and more prolonged than it ought to be, is the first stage and degree. With this topic too are further connected the effects of wines and other fermented liquors upon the brain, as regards both intoxication and sleep; these effects being manifestly related in some part to the action of the kidneys, and varying according to their state in different individuals and under different circumstances.*

Connected closely with the preceding topics is the practical question as to the proportion of sleep best fitted for health, and more especially for the well-being of the sensorial powers. It is obvious that this can be answered explicitly only for individual cases. One temperament undoubtedly requires more than another; nor can the sufficiency of the function be measured merely by number of hours, varying as it does in all that may be termed its intensity and completeness. The remarks, already made, clearly point out these distinctions, to which the mind and body have equal and similar relation.

The effects of deficiency of sleep are more familiar to us than those which belong to its habitual excess. Yet this excess, as a habit, may unquestionably exist. The brain may be kept too long, at each successive period of sleep, in a state which, though strictly speaking as natural as waking, is equally liable to be unduly extended; and

* In Dr. Christison's work on Granular Degeneration of the Kidneys, there are many important remarks on the connexion of these organs with the diseases of the brain.

which, as we have seen, may pass into disease by gradations scarcely to be defined. The expressions of Aretæus,
ὑπνος πολλος παχυτης, αργιη, ομιχλη της αισθησιος· and
again, ὑπνος πολυς ναρκᾳ τας αισθησιας τῆς κεφαλης· are
just in every part of their application. For the state of
the sensorium produced by excess of sleep, appears in a
strict sense, to be one unfavourable to its powers of perception and action. Such state may, with some fitness, be
described as a chronic disorder of the brain; affecting more
or less all the functions of the body, but particularly those
of animal life. It belongs to old age, as an effect of
natural changes, and a part of the dispensation of human
existence. But the growth of habit and self-indulgence
may prematurely bring it on; and the physician is bound
to have regard to this contingency, as well as to the opposite condition of sleep deficient in amount.*

It would appear that, independently of any abridgment
of proper rest, there is something of ill effect to the brain
in the sudden interruption of sleep, often repeated. Whatever the physical difference of the states of sleep and
waking, it seems that the change from the former to the
latter ought to be gradual, as are the approaches of sleep
when coming on. The action of the heart is generally
quickened, or otherwise disturbed, by such interruption.
The same emotion of mind occurs as from any sudden
surprise; and not unfrequently there is a painful and difficult effort in recovering the entire consciousness of the
waking state.

---

* Ὑπνος, αγρυπνιη, αμφοτερα του μετριου μαλλον γενομενα, κακον.—*Hip-
pocrat. Aphorism.* The "vigilans stertit" of the Satirist describes
what is often a reality in life.

Among the causes which influence sleep and dreaming, I doubt whether changes in the state of the atmosphere have been sufficiently noticed. My attention having been casually drawn to this point some years ago, I have since made many observations upon it; and with more uniformity of result than could be expected, seeing the many other causes which act concurrently—as time, quantity and kind of food; excitement or fatigue of mind or body; habit as to times of sleep; and the variations due to actual disease. Removing these sources of error as far as possible, I have found that any sudden and considerable fall of the barometer produces in many persons a sort of lassitude and drowsiness, followed by restless and uneasy sleep, and frequently a state of laborious dreaming. We may doubt whether this influence depends on changes in the balance of circulation so produced, or on alterations in the electrical state of the air concurring with its change of weight, and thereby affecting certain functions of the nervous system. However this be, I cannot doubt the reality of the fact as one of frequent occurrence. It is indeed merely an example, among so many others, of the partial subjection of the phenomena of life to the agents which are ever in movement around us.*

---

* During the month preceding the time when I am now writing (April, 1836), there have been two or three very singular and sudden depressions of the barometer (one of more than an inch within a few hours, from a point already low), attended by gales of unwonted violence on the southern and western coasts of England. It has occurred to me on all these occasions, but particularly on the latter, to observe similar influence, as respects sleep, on myself and many other persons; selecting for evidence those in ordinary health, rather than such as were suffering under any malady at the time.

CHAP. VI.

ON THE RELATIONS OF DREAMING, INSANITY, ETC.

DREAMING — insanity in its many forms — intoxication from wine or narcotics — and the phenomena arising from cerebral disease, are the four great mines of mental discovery still open to us;—if indeed any thing of the nature of discovery remains, on a subject which has occupied and exhausted the labours of thinking men in all ages. These several states, singly and in their connexion with each other, unfold facts, and illustrate relations, which seemingly could have been known to us from no other source. By the curtailment or suspension of certain functions, by the excess of others, and by the altered balance and connexion of all, a sort of analysis is obtained of the nature of mind, which its waking and healthy acts cannot equally afford, either to individual consciousness or the observation of others.

The following remarks relate chiefly to the states of dreaming and insanity, and come naturally in sequel to the subject of the last chapter. The conditions of delirium, intoxication, and other morbid affections of the sensorium, are all concerned in expounding the same general relations; but more partially and transiently than the former. A treatise on the subject, to be complete, would require full illustration from all.

The relations and resemblances of these several states

are indeed well deserving of note, even in their most
general aspect. A dream put into action (as in reality it
is, under certain conditions of somnambulism) might become madness in one or other of its most frequent forms;
and, conversely, insanity may often with fitness be called
a waking and active dream. Delirium and intoxication
are transient effects, from temporary causes, of that condition of sensorium which, more deeply fixed and longer
continued, obtains the name and produces all the aspects
of mental derangement. It is obvious that there are circumstances in common here, not sufficient indeed to
identify these various states—for how difficult to identify
the several conditions of one only!—but enough to show
that certain analogous changes occur as the cause and
foundation of all.

Insanity, from having the characters of a malady, and
this often of hereditary nature;—from its deep import as
such to all the relations of human life—and from the
strange and painful forms it assumes—has ever been
viewed with more profound interest than any of the states
thus allied to it. The feeling has led physicians and
medical writers of every age to seek intently for some
formal definition of madness—a vain and unprofitable
research! Its shapes and aspects are as various as those of
the human mind in a sound state, and as little to be
defined by any single phrases, however laboriously devised.
Where such definitions are attempted, especially in courts
of law, they fitly become matter of ridicule, or causes of
contradiction and perplexity. Mental derangement, however the name be used, is not one thing, nor can it be
treated as such. It differs in kind not less than in degree;

and in each of its varieties we may often trace through different cases all the gradations between a sound and unsound understanding, on the very points where reason is thus disordered.

The importance of obtaining assured practical tests in this matter cannot be doubted. The object is one which concerns in a thousand ways the welfare of individuals and of society. Amongst the many proposed, in cases of difficult legal discrimination, probably the most certain is the sudden change of habitual judgments, feelings, and actions, without obvious cause. The proof from such change is manifestly more secure than any appeal to an imaginary common standard of reason, which scarcely any two persons would estimate alike. But there are many cases, where, from the small scope of change and its limitation to certain subjects, this criterion cannot be obtained. And instances of the kind just mentioned are in fact more numerous, where mere peculiarities of the mind in its sane state may be followed through successive steps into the gravest forms of mental disorder.

On this latter view we are entitled chiefly to rest in every inquiry as to the nature and causes of insanity. We shall find here a wider and more secure basis on which to found observation, than in any other mode of regarding the subject: and if such phrase were permitted as a "just theory of madness," I know no principle so capable of affording it as that which views all the forms of insanity, including delirium, in their relation to corresponding healthy states of mind; tracing this connexion through those intermediate grades, which are so numerously exposed to us in the various conditions of human existence.

The diversities of the mind in what is accounted its healthy
state; — the effect of passions in suddenly altering its
whole condition, of slighter emotions in gradually changing
it, and of other incidents of life in affecting one or more
particular faculties; — its subjection periodically to sleep,
and casually to the states of intoxication, somnambulism,
and reverie; — its gradual transition in fever from a state
where there is consciousness of vague and wandering ideas
to that of perfect delirium; — all these furnish so many
passages through which we may follow sanity into insanity;
and connect the different forms of disordered intellect,
as well with each other, as with the more natural and
healthy functions of the mind.

Even looking to the broad distinction between congenital idiocy (*amentia*), where there is simple deficiency
of natural faculties; and active insanity (*dementia*) in its
more various and formidable shapes — we find various
connexions between them, best illustrated in those cases
where a more active form of madness subsides by degrees
into fatuity. The complications of the mind in its healthy
state are such; its natural changes so frequent and sudden; its relations to the body so various; and the causes of
disordered action so obscure, that we must be satisfied by
classing the facts generally; without drawing those arbitrary lines which nature does not recognise, and which observation perpetually belies. Still, however, certain general
distinctions are required on this subject; not merely for
the sake of arrangement, but yet more to provide for the
communication and common understanding upon cases,
the right view and treatment of which are so important to
human welfare. Many ingenious and learned physicians

have devoted their attention to this object. Its difficulty is attested by the various methods of classification proposed; each having some peculiar merit, but none, as I think, comprising all the various forms of mental disorder which occur in actual life.*

If it were an object to obtain a description of insanity, which might apply to the greatest number of cases of such disorder, I believe this would be found in the conditions which most associate it with dreaming; viz., the loss, partial or complete, of power to distinguish between unreal images created within the sensorium and the actual perceptions drawn from the external senses, thereby giving to the former the semblance and influence of realities — and secondly, the alteration or suspension of that faculty of mind by which we arrange and associate the perceptions and thoughts successively coming before us.†

Though this general description will by no means apply to all that is termed mental derangement, particularly to the various cases of moral insanity, yet, from the extensive influence of the causes denoted in it, there is much reason for their careful consideration — and particularly as they strikingly illustrate those gradations from the sound to the

---

* The classification of mental disorders adopted by Dr. Prichard may be considered one of the simplest and most exact. That of Esquirol, though founded on the long experience of a most able physician, is scarcely perhaps so precise. I might name other and more recent suggestions on this subject, but all liable to the causes of imperfection noticed above.

† All the varieties which Dr. Arnold has brought under the general terms of *ideal* and *notional* insanity, would seem more or less distinctly referable to the above heads.

I

unsound mind, which I have mentioned as affording the
best basis for every part of this inquiry.

A principal modifying cause, when tracing these relations between insanity and dreaming, will be found in the
varying degree of exclusion of sensations from without.
This exclusion, as we have seen in the last chapter, is not
marked by any single and definite limit, even in what may
be deemed the soundest sleep.   It varies presumably at
every moment of time ; and not only as to the degree in
which the general power of perception is present, but even
as to the ratio of impression from different organs.   One
sense, in the plainest meaning of the expression, may be
more asleep than another.   In dreams this exclusion of
external sensations is generally more complete than in
madness, or the ordinary state of intoxication; and here,
accordingly, the *excursus* of aberration appears to be
widest.   Cicero says, and justly, that if it had been so
ordered by nature that we should actually do in sleep all
we dream, every man would have to be bound down before going to bed : — "majores enim, quam ulli insani,
efficerent motus somniantes."*

Much has been written on the subject of spectral illusions; and not without reason, from their strange and
almost mysterious nature — from the seeming warrant they
give to the wildest tales of credulity — and yet further,
from the link they form in the chain betwixt sound reason
and madness.†   Without repeating instances which have

* De Divinatione, 59.

† In the Zauber Bibliothek, a curious work, by G. C. Horst (1825),
will be found two or three striking narratives to which this interpretation manifestly belongs, though presented here under a more in-
definite and mysterious aspect.

become familiar, I may remark that these singular phenomena — while connected on the one side with dreaming,
delirium, and insanity — are related on the other, by a
series of gradations, with the most natural and healthy
functions of the mind. From the recollected images of
objects of sense, which the volition, rationally exercised,
places before our consciousness for the purposes of thought,
and which the reason duly separates from the realities
around us; we have a gradual transition, under different
states of the sensorium, to those spectral images or illusions which come unbidden into the mind; dominate alike
over the senses and reason; and either by their intensity
or duration, produce disorder in the intellectual functions,
and in all the actions depending thereon.*

In the gradations between these two states the most
remarkable is that in which the images of sensible objects,
having no present reality, do nevertheless intrude themselves so forcibly that they cannot be put aside, although
the person is fully awake, and conscious of the presence of
illusion. Numerous instances of this fact are related. I

---

* In illustration of the strange and complex character of these
phenomena, I would mention a faculty the mind occasionally exercises
of modifying, by a sort of voluntary effort, the spectral images which
come involuntarily before the perception, when the eyes are closed.
An outline or figure, having some likeness to a face, may often by a
certain effort be more closely assimilated to it; and the supplementary features made to stand out, as if at our bidding. This fact I
have often attested in my own case. It is related by Goethe, in his
treatise, *Zur Morphologie und Wissenschaft*, that he had the power of
giving a type, or progressive expansion, to phantasms or images
coming casually before his mind — an expression, doubtless, of the
appearances to which we are here alluding.

have myself met with many remarkable examples of it; and more than one attesting that recorded by Dr. Abercrombie, in which the patient, though creating the illusion by an effort of will, had no equal power of removing it by voluntary effort. I have notes of one singular case, where the patient, a robust young man, a native of Germany, suffering under various symptoms of cerebral disorder, was so severely affected by the continuance of these phantoms of intensely painful kind, and by the associations attending them, that his hair, in the course of about ten weeks, changed its colour from black to a greyish white; of which latter colour it grew again, after being shaved off. Another case, which has more recently come under my care, is rendered interesting by the long duration of the disorder; the tendency to such spectral images, and illusions of hearing concurrent with them, having continued (though with considerable intervals between) for nearly twenty-five years.* In all these examples, we may affirm that the images are furnished solely by the memory of former impressions on the senses; although when reaching the degree of spectral illusions, they probably, like the dreams to which they are closely akin, assume combinations which could not occur in the healthy and waking state.†

* The case of this lady, in a prior part of its history, is related by Sir D. Brewster in his volume on Natural Magic, and well deserves perusal in illustration of this curious subject.

† Aristotle, in his remarkable chapter on Memory, expressly notices these spectral illusions, and characterises clearly the modes in which they are perceived and act on the mind.

Τα γαρ φαντασματα ελεγον ὡς γινομενα, και ὡς μνημονευοντες· τουτο δε γινεται, ὁταν τις την μη εικονα ὡς εικονα θεωρῇ.

It is not difficult to understand how some of the most singular incongruities of madness may arise from this coinage of the brain — this struggle betwixt spectral illusions and actual impressions on the senses ; each severally believed, and each brought to bear upon action. The combination of these conditions is so various, the changes among them often so rapid, as to explain every degree of such mental aberration, as well as the diversity of forms under which they occur; from the simple reverie of the absent man, to the wildest incongruities of the maniac. The former is readily recalled from his transient absorption by incidents or sensations from without. The mind of the latter is engrossed by images, intense enough to compel belief, and to create the emotions and actions which constitute madness. From my own observation I cannot doubt that such causes are of frequent occurrence.

Nor is the application of this view limited to delusions in which sight is concerned. As these images often assume the character of reality, so likewise do the impressions of sound, under certain disordered states of the sensorium, occasionally become such as to excite perfect belief in their

And again, more expressly, when treating of dreams —

Διο και τοῖς πυρεττουσιν ενιοτε φαινεται ζῶα εν τοῖς τοιχοις, απο μικρᾶς ὁμοιοτητος τῶν γραμμων συντιθεμενων· και ταῦτα ενιοτε συνεπιτεινει τοῖς παθεσιν οὗτως, ὡς αν μεν μη σφοδρα καμνωσι, μη λανθανειν ὁτι ψευδος· αν δε μειζον ᾖ το παθος, και κινεισθαι προς αυτα.

The phenomenon, having always existed, could not at any time escape notice. But it is interesting to mark these earlier notices of the fact, especially in the connexion given it with other mental phenomena, by one of the most remarkable observers of any age.

existence from without. The noises of organs, bells,
street cries, and " airy tongues that syllable men's names,"
are known and recorded as frequent forms of these auricu-
lar delusions. Instances are common in cases of insanity,
where the patient is so strongly affected by imagined
voices, as to produce on his part earnest or passionate
rejoinder. I have known these delusions of hearing such,
in a case of delirium tremens, that the patient held a long
and angry colloquy with an imaginary person, whom he
supposed (there being no deception of sight) in an adjoin-
ing room. He allowed pauses to intervene, while his
opponent might be presumed to be speaking; yet, amidst
all this, answered immediately and with correctness every
question I put to himself. In another case of mental
derangement recorded in my notes, the patient held frequent and excited conversations; in which he sometimes
professed to hear the answers given to him; at other times
bore both parts himself, but in different tones of voice for
each of the supposed parties engaged.

These illusions of hearing, like those of vision, may be
traced through every stage — from the imaginations of
sounds created by voluntary effort, or stealing upon us
independently of the will, but felt to be without external
source—to those which possess the mind with entire
belief of their reality, and force it into action founded on
this belief. A familiar example of what may be termed
the first stage of insubordination to the will, is that of certain musical sounds or airs coming unsought for upon the
attention, and even tormenting it by their persistence,
despite every effort to put them aside. This illustration
is made still more curious by the fact that a musical air,—

thus hanging, as it were, upon the ear of the mind, — may be wholly suspended for half-an-hour (as I have often found from my own experience) by some more urgent demand on the attention, yet suddenly recur when this cause is removed.   Harsh sounds long continued, as of a carriage during a day's journey, will frequently continue to make similar though feebler impressions upon the sensorium, for hours afterwards.   Some of these cases may depend upon changes within the organ of hearing itself: others, from their nature, must clearly be referred to the sensorium or percipient part.   As this class of delusions has been altogether less noted than the preceding, I subjoin two or three singular cases which I find among my notes.   They illustrate more particularly the gradations of state just alluded to, and the connexion between a natural and healthy function and the morbid actions of the same part.*

---

* Mr. ——, at the age of eighty-five, in a feeble bodily frame, preserved a clear and acute understanding, great powers of humour, and a deep interest in all passing events. No affection of the brain had ever occurred in the course of life. A casual fall, on the 19th of May, threw his head with some violence against the edge of a sofa: a swelling was raised on the forehead, but no other obvious injury: some faintness ensued, but no stupor or sickness. An hour or two afterwards there came on a failure both in the memory and articulation of words. He could not remember the names of his servants, nor, when wishing to express his wants to them, could he find the right words to do so. The sounds he uttered, in seeking for speech, were not only unintelligible to others, but *consciously so to himself;* a singularity he reasoned upon at the time, and perfectly recollected afterwards.

A restless night, with some vomiting, ensued; but the following day the memory and speech returned to their usual state, and continued free from disorder on the 21st. On the 22d, when driving out

We have instances, chiefly in cases of actual insanity, of corresponding illusions of the sense of touch, scarcely

in his carriage, for the first time after the accident, there came on the singular *lusus* of two voices, seemingly close to the ear — in rapid dialogue, or rather repetition of phrases, unconnected with any event of present occurrence, and almost without meaning. Mr. —— described himself as perfectly conscious of the fallacy of this, but as wholly unable to check or withdraw the perception of these voices, or to change the phrases they seemed to utter. There was no nervousness on his part, but rather amusement in the strangeness of the phenomenon, and the absurdity of the speeches to which he felt himself listening. The same state continued during dinner. In the evening, while seeking to read, similar voices seemed to accompany him, as if reading aloud — sometimes getting on a few words in advance, but not beyond what the eye might have reached — sometimes substituting totally different words; the whole having the effect of distinct speech from without, and being entirely beyond the control of his will.

These symptoms (of which I have notes made at the moment by Mr. —— himself) were almost wholly removed the next day, and never afterwards recurred. Their relation to some of the conditions of dreaming will be obvious; the main difference being the presence of that waking consciousness which receives real sensations from without, and regulates the course of thoughts within.

In another interesting case which occurred to me, there was a well marked passage from the state in which the patient (a gentleman about fifty-two, without any obvious disease), believed in and acted upon the reality of such illusive sounds and conversations, to the condition in which, having still similar sensations, he recognised and treated them as delusions. The first state, which lasted many months, had the character of partial derangement, and was necessarily treated as such. I saw him both at this time, and soon after the change to the second state. On the latter occasion, I inquired how, when the same articulate sounds still seemed present, he had learnt to regard them as delusions? He told me it was partly by his never discovering any person in the places whence the voices had come; chiefly by finding himself able on trial to suggest the words which were thus seemingly uttered by some one external to himself. To these reasons

less remarkable than those of sight and hearing. Even
the senses of taste and smell furnish various intimations of

might doubtless have been added some change in the actual state of
the brain, however incomprehensible its nature and cause.

I may notice further respecting this case, that there was for the
most part some obvious foundation in the thoughts or feelings at the
time for the phrases which seemed to reach the ear from without.
This fact abounds in curious inferences. It appears to make a breach
for the time in the identity of the rational being. We have the
strange phenomenon before us of thoughts and emotions rising within
the mind, and arranged in the phraseology of words; which words,
however, by some morbid perversion of the functions of the brain,
are received and believed by the consciousness as coming from persons
without. It is, if such expression be allowed, a sort of duplicity of
the mind in its dealing with itself. Cases of this nature have kindred
with some of the curious phenomena of somnambulism and trance.
The madman of Horace, also, will be recollected here, —

> " Qui se credebat miros audire tragœdos,
> In vacuo lætus sessor plausorque theatro."—*Epist.* II. 2. 129.

In a third case, a lady advanced in years, and much devoted to
music throughout life, became subject without obvious cause to
impressions of musical sounds or airs, so unceasing, and often of such
intensity, as greatly to fatigue and distress her, and even seriously to
interfere with nightly rest. Of the tunes thus impressing her with a
sort of reality, some were familiar to her, others altogether new combinations. Sometimes the sounds were harsher and more irregular,
yet still tending to assume musical time. She made distinctions between two kinds of sounds; some heard as if from without, others again
as if within the head. The struggle between the voluntary power
conscious of the delusion, and the physical sensations, offered many
curious facts. A particular air could generally be brought on by the
will, but not dismissed again, except by a strong effort to take up
another. When the attention was closely given to any particular
tune, the notes were often hurried on violently; or the tune came
suddenly to a close, the consciousness taking it up again from the beginning; this hurry and sudden change being always a cause of
increased distress to the patient. There was no pain of the head in

similar kind. Hysterical affections, which, when highly aggravated, may be said to stand on the brink of insanity, abound in these examples of disordered or illusive perceptions of touch, pain, and other feelings—very difficult even for the patients themselves to define; but which result from internal causes affecting all parts of the nervous system.

This struggle then, occurring in every form and degree, betwixt illusive and real sensations, affords perhaps the widest basis on which to reason as to some of the most frequent hallucinations of insanity. While explaining the connexion of these phenomena with dreaming and reverie, it indicates a foundation for the whole in that natural function of mind by which we perpetually change our relation to external objects, even when all the senses are open and awake; — at one moment abstracting our consciousness from them altogether — at another, admitting some sensations, while others are excluded; — these unceasing changes, which in their series make up the chain or circle of life, being sometimes the effect of the will, sometimes wholly beyond its control. On this subject, which has such important connexion with all the mental functions, intellectual and moral, in health and

---

this case. Deafness, though not to great extent, came on concurrently with the affection just described. The only other symptoms were some unsteadiness in walking, and occasional intermission of pulse. I saw the lady at intervals for a period of some months, during which time no material change occurred in her state. She died two or three years afterwards.

In none of these cases was there spectral illusion; the voices and sounds being unassociated with any visual image. Though the two illusions occasionally co-exist, I believe this to occur but rarely.

in disease, I have spoken at large in a preceding chapter
of this Volume.

Though we thus find foundation for many kinds of insanity even in a natural law of our constitution, more is
required to explain the strange incongruities of thought
which occur in these cases of delusion, as well as in others
where no false impressions on the senses exist. We cannot
perhaps go further than to affirm, as matter of observation,
that the same changes, whatsoever they be, which impair
the power of distinguishing between deceptive images and
the realities of sense, do also impair that faculty of rightly
combining and recalling ideas (μνημη ξυνθετικη) upon
which the condition of man, as a rational being, depends.
Here, as I have before observed, the relation to the state
of sleep and dreaming is most distinctly marked.   Let any
one close his eyes, when in easy posture and quiet place ;
no strong impressions acting on the external senses.
While yet retaining enough of waking consciousness to
note the fact, images will be felt to steal upon realities,
and ideas to blend more confusedly together, with less
power of retaining them, or regulating their succession.
A slight disturbance may recall the mind for a moment to
itself; which being removed, it lapses again into the same
state.   This, carried further, becomes dreaming.   The
access to one sense is now almost closed; the capacity of
receiving impressions from the others impaired; the powers
of volition diminished and misdirected ; the consciousness
of personal identity, essential as an exponent of reason in
its sound state, lost or greatly obscured.

Let a similar state of sensorium exist from other causes,
and for a longer time, but leaving free the action of the

external senses and the power of volition, and we have a condition scarcely to be distinguished from many forms of mental derangement. Images and perceptions, real and unreal, co-exist and confuse each other; while actions result from both. From the same physical causes, presumably, the trains of thought become disordered, and ordinary associations are changed; or if they be in part coincident with the natural state, that power at least is lessened of retaining them before the mind as objects of thought, which seems an essential part of our rational existence. And as these causes, whatever their nature, may easily be conceived to affect one part of the sensorium more than another, and to vary in degree at different times, we have in such diversities the explanation,—not indeed of the proximate cause,—but of the relations of many of the most singular and anomalous forms of mental derangement.

I have just noticed the confusion as to personal identity which so often occurs in dreams, producing some of their strangest anomalies and aberrations. It is well worthy of note, in reference to the connexion between the two states, how often a similar confusion forms part of the more fixed hallucinations of insanity. Examples to this effect abound in medical works, and are familiar to the experience of every physician. The momentary aberrations of the dream become the more lasting and active delusions of madness.

The approaches of delirium in fever well illustrate many of these phenomena; often exhibiting, within an hour or two, every grade from perfect reason to a state of wild or furious perversion of mind. First, the wandering images

or thoughts, which yet are known to be unreal, and frequently described by the patient himself as *nonsense* —
then, the vague rambling talk; from which, however, the
patient is still disengaged by being spoken to, by alteration
of posture, or other excitement—afterwards, under further
but gradual change, the state of perfect delirium, where
every function of the mind is disordered by the unreal
images and false combinations which possess it, uncon-
trolled by impressions from without.

In the last chapter I have spoken at length on that
rational theory of sleep, by which it is regarded as a series
of ever-fluctuating states; varying not only in general
intensity, but even more remarkably in the degree in
which different mental functions are under its influence at
the same moment of time. This view, which more happily
than any other explains the various aspects of sleep and
dreaming, is that also which we may best follow in reasoning upon their connexion with permanent states of mental
disorder.

In many points, indeed, the phenomena both of dreaming
and insanity find more illustration from the waking moods
of mind than is generally supposed. Dreams appear in-
consecutive in the series of impressions and thoughts which
compose them; and are so in fact in different degrees,
according to the varying condition of sleep. But let any
one follow with consciousness or immediate recollection
the ramblings and transitions of the waking state, when
the mind is not bound down to any one subject, and no
strong impressions are present to the senses — and he will
often find these no less singular, abrupt, and rapid in
change; though the effect of such irregularity is here

subordinate to certain regulating causes, which are absent during sleep.

The admission of external sensations is amongst the most important of these. Their influence in correcting aberrant trains of thought is marked in numerous familiar instances; still more remarkably when causes of actual disorder are present. A person on the verge of intoxication feels confusion of thought rapidly coming on him when he closes his eyes, which is lessened or removed when opening them again; and such alternation may repeatedly occur. A patient under low rambling delirium will often pause from this when a question is asked him, or when any distinct impression is made on the senses; relapsing almost instantly again into the same state. Examples of this kind show how slight the line is, if line there be, which separates the healthy actions of mind from those of morbid nature.*

In children, where the corrections from reason and experience are less complete than in adults, dreams often assume a very singular aspect in their passage to the waking state. I have seen cases, where a child, waking affrighted by some imaginations of an unquiet dream, has continued for an hour or longer in state of agitation

---

* Milton, in a fine passage (though perhaps somewhat too abstruse for his occasion), describes this vague imagery of the mind, when Reason has retired to Nature's rest : —

> " Oft in her absence mimic Fancy wakes
> To imitate her ; but, misjoining shapes,
> Wild work produces oft, and most in dreams ;
> Ill matching words and deeds long past or late."
>
> *Paradise Lost*, Book V

resembling delirium; the unreal images or ideas still possessing the mind, and being only slowly removed by actual impressions on the senses. Even in adults, we know by experience that the last images of an excited dream often hang painfully and perplexingly on the mind, when awake again to external objects; and that we reason and feel upon them, before fully convinced of their unreality. I may add, further, a remarkable fact — strongly attested to us, though not free from ambiguity — viz., that the images created by a dream are sometimes actually seen as such by a person suddenly opening his eyes on waking; resembling, in fact, those spectral images seen on other occasions, to which we have already adverted.* All such phenomena illustrate well the particular relations we are now seeking to examine.

Another connexion between these several states is that afforded by the curious phenomena of reverie, trance, or cataleptic ecstasy; where, with the external senses as much closed as in perfect sleep, it would seem that the intellectual and voluntary powers are sometimes exercised much more clearly and consecutively, yet not under the same relation to consciousness and memory, as in the

---

* Müller notices this phenomenon, and expresses his conviction of it on his own experience. (Ueber die phantastiischen Gesichter-scheinungen.) He mentions, farther, that the same observation had occurred long before to Spinoza. Every one may find occasion to make the trial for himself, with allowance for those circumstances which may vary or annul the results—such as the different intensity of the images of the dream, the interval of time before the eyes are opened, and possibly also the temperament of the individual. I am not sure that I ever recognised the appearance in my own case.

waking state. Though the evidence as to these extraordinary cases is much obscured by fiction, there is quite
enough that is authentic to give them place among the
most remarkable forms of sensorial disorder. Here, however, we may still follow out the connexion with the more
common phenomena of mind. Reverie, in this medical
sense, is but a higher degree of that which we call such in
ordinary language; or what is still more usually termed
absence of mind. And this again is merely the excess of
the condition, common to all and of constant occurrence,
in which the consciousness is detached for a time from
objects of sense actually present to the organs, concentrating itself upon trains of thought and feeling within;—
a condition which belongs to and characterises man as
an intellectual being.

I can scarcely doubt that to some of the states just
described we must refer the mesmeric sleep or trance, of
which I have spoken in the last chapter. The effect,
though more striking from the means being less familiar,
is, as we have seen, but one of the many modifications the
mind undergoes even in its healthy state. The facts
stated above show further by close analogy, how speech,
or even partial conversations, may occur during these
trances. But as regards the purport of the speech so
uttered, much of what we find recorded by the mesmerists
must be set down to chance or credulity; as nothing but
direct miraculous interposition could explain that which is
proffered to our belief.

In extreme old age, again, the phenomena of dreaming
and waking aberration are still more closely blended together. The two states of sleep and waking are severally

more imperfect in kind; the distinction betwixt them becomes less marked; and the whole of mental existence seems as if contracted from both sides into a narrower space, and a lower scale of intensity. I have known instances of this kind, where, without any obvious disease of the vital organs, life had become a vague and feeble dream; scarcely broken into periods of time; and with the capacity almost lost of distinguishing between the real and unreal images which flitted unconnectedly before the mind. These cases, which cannot be looked upon without deep interest, undoubtedly depend upon physical changes taking place in the brain; enfeebling and confusing all relations with the external world, and the associations and actions thereon depending.

There is greater difficulty in reasoning on the condition of the mind in infancy; yet this has doubtless its relation to the succeeding parts of life, and especially, as it would appear, to the cases where the intellect is disordered or permanently deficient. Idiotcy, if congenital sometimes, seems in other instances to be simply an arrest of the natural course and progress of the functions. The sensorial idiot retains the infant mind in an adult body. But as these functions may be thus morbidly checked at some point in their growth, so may they also, from physical causes, revert from a more advanced state to one of earlier life; and frequent examples occur, where both the deficiencies and hallucinations of insanity show close resemblance to the unformed intellect and character of the child. This connexion abounds in curious inferences, and well deserves further examination of its details.

I need scarcely dwell upon the application of the pre-

K

ceding remarks to the effects of alcohol and other narcotic substances, in their different modes of action on the brain. The states thereby produced are exceedingly various; for even intoxication, commonly so termed, differs greatly in kind as well as in degree. In one man it is the condition of a maniac — in another, the stupid oppression of all the faculties of thought and action. Still it will be found, upon close observation, that these various states all graduate more or less distinctly into one another; and that they are connected in common with the phenomena of insanity and dreaming — not merely by vague resemblances of external aspect, but yet more by analogous changes in the sensorium itself; in its relation to external objects through the senses, and in those combinations within, which constitute trains of thought and become the causes of disordered action.

While seeking thus to associate together various states of mental aberration in the intellectual functions, and to illustrate thereby the nature of each, it were vain to push inquiry far into the proximate cause of these phenomena. That changes, partial or general, transient or permanent, occur in the nervous substance of the brain, producing such conditions, is rendered certain by various evidence.*

---

* Sir W. Ellis, in his Treatise on Insanity, has stated, in evidence of the structural causes of this disorder, that out of 221 cases, male and female, examined after death, not fewer than 207 afforded proof of disease either in the brain or its membranes. It must be added, however, that the reports of Esquirol and Pinel are much below this estimate; and there is reason to doubt whether, in drawing it up, sufficient attention has been given to discriminate between the morbid

The most distinct proof, independently of that from actual observation, is furnished by hereditary insanity; which, however ignorant we may be of the particular structure affected, must doubtless be produced by some organisation disposing to the disease, or to the series of changes which evolve it. This subject of predisposition is one we are bound to keep in view in all researches and reasoning on the subject; not, indeed, as affording any certain knowledge (for hereditary transmission is itself a profound mystery throughout), but as checking hasty or partial conclusions drawn from other sources.

How far the changes producing different forms of insanity depend on the quantity of blood in the brain— on its local distribution — on the rate or manner of circulation — or on the varying qualities of the blood itself, — are inquiries of much interest and great difficulty. The history of all cerebral disease, and the examination of those instances where it has been fatal, show the remarkable influence of these several conditions; and particularly how small an amount of obvious change in the circulation, as in the slighter degrees of inflammation of the membranes, is capable of producing great disturbance in the mental functions. But still this is an influence only of indirect kind. Even in what seem the simpler of the cases before us — those of dreaming, intoxication, or the

changes taking place immediately before death, and those of earlier date, which may more probably have been concerned as causes of insanity. The liability to error from this source is obvious in its nature, and requires to be guarded against in every part of pathology and morbid anatomy.

delirium of fever — we must look to the nervous substance as the immediate source of the remarkable changes
taking place. Its alterations, however produced, or in
whatsoever consisting, are the causes which lie before us
for discovery. But whether our present methods of research, or others yet to be devised, may hereafter afford us
more complete knowledge, it is impossible to affirm.

While pursuing, indeed, our inquiry into the physical
causes of insanity, it is important to define, as exactly as
possible, what is the right course, and what the pre-
sumable limit of discovery. In ascertaining the effects of
altered circulation of blood through the brain, be it excess
or deficiency, we are fixing a very important class of facts,
and of great practical value. They are further of especial
interest to the mode of viewing insanity which I seek at
present to inculcate ; inasmuch as it seems certain from
observation that the first effect of these changes of circulation is simply to excite or depress, without altering the
nature of the functions in the parts thus affected. In
slight inflammation, for example, of the upper surface of
the brain, we find an unwonted irritation and restlessness
of mind, excesses of natural temper, and a want of self-
control ; all which effects may terminate here, the inflammation being subdued. Or in cases of simple excited
circulation, such as may be induced by mental emotion or
by stimulants taken internally, but below the level of
inflammatory action or intoxication, we often find an
excitement of the faculties and feelings, which may be
deemed the first step of deviation from the natural state.
These early degrees of change are frequently the source
whence discovery may best be derived.

Still, as I have remarked above, this influence of the circulation, in relation to the intellectual functions, is wholly subordinate to the changes in the state of the nervous substance which intervene. We have gained a step, but it is only a step, to something beyond. And the same remark applies to alterations in the quality of the blood; whether consisting in different degrees of arterialization, or in the admission of substances foreign to its composition. From the nature of these causes, they have a diffused influence upon the intimate structure of the brain, by which certain of the sensorial functions are occasionally suspended altogether. Local congestions or extravasations of blood—serous effusions into the ventricles or between the membranes — thickenings of the cranium, or irregularities of its inner surface — morbid deposits or tumours within the brain — abscesses in its substance — these and other deviations from natural structure, whether congenital or from disease, may be classed as causes affecting parts of the nervous substance, and suggesting inquiry into the relation between these parts and the particular faculty or function affected in each case. But they do not carry our knowledge further.

The question then ultimately and necessarily brings us to the changes in the nervous structure itself; thus variously acted upon by external causes, and producing in effect such remarkable alteration in the mental functions. The two morbid states of softening and induration of the brain, and its deficient development as to size, either in the whole or parts of its structure, seem to be some approach to a solution; and yet, if rightly estimated, lead us very little way towards it.* Not that we are to disregard such results of examination, as the medullary substance being softer than natural, or the cineritious substance darker. These alterations, though slight perhaps in degree, are presumably, from their nature and diffusion, more effective for permanent change and injury of function than many which are more obvious to remark. Looking indeed to what we know of the delicate and complex structure of some parts of the nervous system of the brain — to the impossibility of tracing the texture of other parts by the most minute research—and still more to the nature of the functions to which this system so closely ministers, — we must admit it as likely that the changes going on here, both in health and disease, will in great part be ever hidden from our knowledge. As these actions, however, subtle and eyanescent though they be, are still physical in their nature, the inquiry is one fairly open to us. But it should be so conducted as not to grasp at partial facts and hasty conclusions, where truth lies at such depth below the surface.

Again, if the states of dreaming, intoxication, and delirium occur and pass away, without leaving traces behind on the brain, we may reasonably conclude that various forms of insanity, which we have seen to be so closely related to them, may exist, and even long continue, without permanent alterations of structure, or changes appreciable by the human eye. That organic differences

* Meckel remarks, what doubtless is true, that in the brain the faults of conformation by defect are much more numerous and important than those by excess.

are often present as an original cause, must be presumed from the cases where the disorder is hereditary in the habit; and from the numerous instances where examination after death shows deviation from the natural structure. But even where there is proof that such organic changes have occurred, and that the derangement depends upon them, it is remarkable to what extent amelioration may for a time take place in the mental symptoms, though the original causes continue the same. Hence we obtain further proof that the proximate cause resides in some parts of structure to which our present means afford us no access, and that to this we must chiefly look for the various fluctuations of the disease.*

Viewing the question more generally, and in reference to the total mass of the brain, it may be stated as probable that where the intellectual and moral functions are those disordered, any physical disease therewith connected will be found to exist in the cerebral hemispheres; con-

---

* I recollect a case of mental derangement, where the post-mortem examination showed great organic changes in the brain; many of them, from their nature, obviously of long standing, and upon which it was next to certain that the symptoms depended. Yet in this instance there occurred not long before death a lucid interval, so far complete and prolonged, as to afford hopes of recovery where none had before existed, and where the event proved that none could reasonably be entertained. Other similar cases I find in my notes, The instances indeed are frequent and familiar, where the memory, affected manifestly, and it may be said permanently, by organic changes in the brain, does nevertheless at intervals, and without obvious cause, recover itself for a moment with singular clearness — then pass suddenly under a cloud as before. An example of this, as it occurred in one of the most eminent men of his time, can never be lost to my remembrance.

sisting either in imperfect original development; or in softening or induration of substance; or in some more especial and local disease of structure. Our actual knowledge scarcely carries us beyond this; though some eminent physiologists have held the opinion that the cineritious neurine of the brain is the particular part related to these functions, and the subject of the diseases which affect them. Every part, indeed, of this topic offers large scope to speculation. In another chapter I have ventured a suggestion as to the effect upon the mental functions of an unequal or incongruous action of the two hemispheres of the brain. As the variety of the disorder presumes a corresponding difference in its cause, another suggestion may arise, whether certain kinds of insanity be not the effect of simple excess or deficiency in quantity of that power (nervous, sensorial, or however denominated) by which the mutual relations of mind and body are maintained? It is certain that such variation as to quantity exists;—certain also that it produces much influence on both these parts of our existence. If we might suppose that some maniacal disorders depend on a morbid excess of this power, we should have an example of the case alluded to above, viz. derangement of mind proceeding from physical causes, but these involving only transient alteration in a natural function, and not any changes of structure which can leave permanent traces behind.

Throughout the whole of the foregoing remarks I have used the term insanity in its most comprehensive sense; seeking to define its varieties chiefly by their relation to the healthy functions of mind; or to other states of mental aberration, either natural like dreaming, or otherwise frequent and familiar to us. It is one of those subjects in which the facts are so complicated, that truth may expediently be sought for simply by varying their arrangement. And this truth is likely to be best obtained when we can thus associate together the natural and morbid conditions by a series of intermediate steps, which bring no new element into our theory of mind, and at the same time render some explanation of the strange and seemingly anomalous variety of these cases. Such gradations are most easily followed in all that regards illusions of the senses. But though becoming less obvious as we advance into the inward recesses of thought, and seek for explanation of those states in which false combinations of ideas, and perverted passions and feelings, are chiefly concerned, yet we may still obtain illustration from the healthy habitudes of mind, especially as seen in the intermediate phenomena of dreaming and intoxication.

In the most complete degree of melancholia, for example, it is often but the exaggeration and persistence of that gloomy mood of mind, which in one degree or another occurs occasionally to every person, overshadowing for the time all the thoughts and feelings of life. This may be the delusion of an hour, readily removed by change of place, occupation, or events. But it may continue longer under the character of hypochondriasis; or become permanent as a form of insanity; still depending on some common cause, however different the intensity and manner of operation.

The most difficult part of the subject, undoubtedly, and that which we can least solve by any knowledge we possess,

is what has been termed Moral, in contradistinction to
Intellectual Insanity; — where no actual false perceptions
exist, and the intellect in its ordinary sense is compara-
tively little affected; but where the feelings, temper, and
habits are vitiated and variously perverted; sometimes
assuming a character very opposite to that of the same
mind in its healthy state, and seeming to alter the whole
moral condition of the being.

It is needless to dwell upon the melancholy details of
cases, which are so familiar to common experience. The
attempt, moreover, is almost painful, of seeking explanation or analogy for them in the more natural conditions of
human character. Yet such relations exist, and may be
easily recognised in particular examples. In truth, we
seldom meet with instances where this moral derangement
is altogether of sudden occurrence, or wholly detached from
the prior life and habits of the individual. It comes upon
the mind gradually, though often very unequally; — sometimes shown at first in the excess or misdirection of certain
accustomed feelings; — these aberrations fostered often by
the very circumstances they create, acquiring the force of
habits, and in the same proportion losing the control of the
intellect and will. The understanding, indeed, though ex-
empt perhaps from common hallucinations, is really perverted or enfeebled in most of these cases, and no longer gives
that direction and balance which is essential to the healthy
state of the mind. Even where a particular feeling or
affection seems changed into one utterly opposite, a closer
view will often show some relation to the previous temperament. While a more general contemplation of human
character will afford the proof that opposite extremes are

not always so distinct or incongruous, as at first sight they may appear.

All wonted methods of delineating character are, indeed, in some sort covenanted and artificial, and scarcely according with the reality of facts. We describe it as a unity, distinctly marked for each individual;—and, in a common sense, this is just. But there are few in whom the feelings and sentiments which compose it do not undergo fluctuations; as well under the influence of age and the more momentous events of life, as also more variously and incessantly from changes that belong to the day or hour; — the conditions of health or sickness — the bodily sensations or instincts — the incidents of social and domestic life — and the many other events which crowd upon every part of existence. Who has not recognised, from experience, the singular disparity between the feelings and imaginations which haunt the hours of wakefulness in the night, and those which exist on the same subjects during the active moments of the day? — or the difference of state under fasting and exhaustion, and after food and rest? — or even from a gleam of sunshine breaking out after cloud and storm? Amidst momentary changes of this kind, particularly in persons of a certain temperament, we may often recognise the elements of those future and more fixed aberrations to which the name of mental derangement is needfully applied. The greater or less facility, indeed, of being thus affected, forms one of the most essential circumstances in character itself; and in few respects do individuals differ more widely than in their power of preserving rational habits, steady and unimpaired, under the circumstances ever pressing upon them. The highest ex-

altation of man lies in this direction; and the state of
mind, moreover, which gives greatest security against
every form of derangement.

The intellectual, as well as moral part of our nature, is
subject to the same continual change; subordinate, it is
true, to the individual faculties of each, but well marked
to common consciousness and observation. Thinking is
not a single or uniform act even in the most sober and
regulated understandings. It varies continually in rapidity
and intensity, according to the conditions of the body, or
influences from without; and the amount of variation,
great in the same person, becomes more obvious when the
observation is directed to many. There are times and
causes which raise the intensity of thought almost to the
condition of a passion, despite every effort to suspend what
is felt to be a morbid and painful state of mind.

These considerations, which might be pursued to much
greater extent, obviously apply to the singular forms of
madness which the French physicians have named Monomania; where we may generally discover connexion with
some more ordinary states of mind; furnishing analogy, at
least, in default of other solution. Most persons have felt
at one time or other (oftenest, as we have seen, during the
" severa silentia noctis ") some dominant idea or feeling to
possess the fancy; retaining its hold with a sort of malig-
nant power, despite all efforts to shake it off; and by degrees distorting the subject, especially if it be a painful
one, into a thousand false and alarming shapes. If this
train of thought be interrupted; and time, society, and
other objects come in between; the mind is felt as if
passing out of a bad dream, which for a while had over-

shadowed it. But let there be a cause for the continuance of this state (and the duration of the impression is at least as explicable as its original occurrence), and we have an approach to monomania in some of its various shapes; nothing apparently wanting but that intensity, which is often so singularly testified in these cases by the actions induced, and by the length of period during which the delusion remains in force. Pinel, one of the best authorities on this subject, mentions instances where the same single insane impression continued without change for twenty or thirty years.*

In fact, the long persistence of the mind in one idea or feeling, not duly broken in upon or blended with others, is a state always leading towards aberration: and a common evidence of insanity, especially in its earlier stage, is that drawn from the predominance of a single impression, faulty perhaps only in the absence of those which should modify and correct it. It may be alleged that this reasoning tends to remove all distinction betwixt the sound and unsound mind; and to reflect madness back, as it were, upon the healthy and natural state of the faculties of man. But this is not truly so. The extremes are widely apart,

---

* It must be admitted that these partial hallucinations, occurring often without obvious cause from without, and holding thus tenaciously on the mind, furnish argument to the phrenologists; and a reasonable one, as far as respects the opinion that there is a plurality of parts about the brain having connexion with different intellectual and moral functions. But phrenology, as I have noticed in another chapter, points out no actual structure in the brain having especial correspondence with these functions, either in healthy or diseased state; and its indications from the form of the cranium are not yet authentic enough to be admitted as a system of facts.

and offer marks of practical distinction which can rarely be misunderstood. The existence of more doubtful cases, such as graduate between reason and insanity, is but a part of that law of continuity which pervades so generally every part of creation. It is attested by the actual difficulty experienced in dealing either legally or morally with these cases; and by the observation of their progress, as well when first passing the limit of reason, as when re-entering it in the course of recovery.

Such observations, and founded on this basis, are the more important, as they bear directly upon every question of treatment. No principle of practice in mental disorders can probably be successful which does not recognise their relation to the phenomena of mind in its healthy state; and some of the most remarkable cures I have known, where physical causes of the infirmity did not exist, have been effected really, if not professedly, by a discreet application of this method. It is not my present purpose to speak on the treatment of these disorders; but I am persuaded this will be found true as a general remark. And equally so the assertion, that from no other source can suggestions be drawn of equal value in the prevention of them, when the predisposition exists in the habit.

Though the subject does not readily admit of separation, yet having chiefly had it in view to illustrate the connexion of insanity in its different forms with the more natural conditions of the mind, I shall not add much as to the immediate causes of this malady. The effects of various kinds of mental and physical excitement, whether with or without hereditary disposition, have so often been discussed, that it is unnecessary here to dwell upon them. They may chiefly be comprised under the several heads of anxiety, distress of circumstances, undue religious excitement, blighted hopes or affections, intemperance, and excessive or deficient use of the natural powers.* There is one point, however, connected with the subject, to which, as having been less noticed, I will shortly allude before closing this chapter.

It seems probable that certain cases of madness depend on a cause which can scarcely exist, even in slight degree, without producing some mental disturbance; viz. the too frequent and earnest direction of the mind inwards upon itself; — the concentration of the consciousness too long continued upon its own functions. It would appear (if we may venture so to surmise) a design in the creation of this wonderful existence which we call soul, that while safely using the faculties given to us in exploring every part of the world of nature without, we should be unable to sustain these powers when directed inwards to the source and centre of their own operations. In this matter every one may make experiments for himself. I believe it will be found that any strong and continuous effort of will to concentrate the mind upon its own workings — to analyse them by consciousness — or even to fix, check, or suddenly change the trains of thought, — is generally followed by speedy and painful confusion, com-

* The recent publications of Dr. Brigham, of Boston, on the influence of mental cultivation and excitement upon health, communicate some singular facts as to the effects produced by commercial, political, and religious excitement in the United States. The proportion of persons deranged in mind to the whole population is, according to his statement, nearly three times as great as in England.

pelling in no long time the abandonment of the act. Even a simple difficulty of recollection, where the mind intently concentrates itself in inward search after some of its own former operations, becomes painful when long continued; and thought is often lost in utter confusion.* I doubt not that the long continuance or frequent repetition of such circumstances, from whatever cause, is sufficient to produce a temporary derangement in minds already predisposed to the infirmity. I have myself known more than one instance of aberration of intellect, which I had every reason to believe thus produced.

These, however, may be termed excesses in the employment of a faculty which it is given us to use. The actual power thus to inquire into the mind and regulate the trains of thought, exists, and is capable of wide and various cultivation. All the greater qualities of intellect lie in this direction, and are associated with the exercise of this faculty. But I do not dwell further on these points, having already discussed them in a former chapter, devoted more especially to the subject.

---

* When speaking elsewhere of the effects of mental attention on the bodily organs, I have noticed these peculiar effects of the continued concentration of the mind upon itself.

CHAP. VII.

ON THE MEMORY, AS AFFECTED BY AGE AND DISEASE.

THIS title includes some of the most curious phenomena which come under the notice of the physician — closely related to those discussed in the preceding chapter, but offering new and equally difficult questions to our inquiry. Even those hypotheses, which, under vague general terms, seem to carry us some steps further than the common understanding of the subject, are wholly at fault in seeking to solve them. And the metaphysician, who is here treading on the same ground with the physiologist and physician, equally fails of reaching any conclusion which can be admitted within the pale of exact science.

A case of slight paralytic affection is at this time before me, where the perceptions from the senses are unimpaired; the memory of persons and events seemingly correct; the intelligence only slightly affected; the bodily functions, though feeble in power, not otherwise disordered; but where the memory of words for speech is so nearly gone, that only the single monosyllable " yes" remains as the sole utterance of all that the patient desires to express. Even when a simple negative is obviously intended, no other word is used. — In another case of recent occurrence, where, in sequel to a paralytic attack two years before, the memory of words had been greatly confused and im-

L

paired, I found them all regained and brought into right use, except the pronouns; which were almost invariably displaced and substituted one for another. — In a third case, where the patient, affected with hemiplegia at a very advanced age, passed into a state of low rambling delirium a few days before his death; all that he uttered, whether in answer or otherwise, was in French, — a language he had not been known to speak at any time for thirty years before. This continued until his utterance ceased to be intelligible altogether.

I cite these cases merely as examples, recently present to myself, of the numberless others in which this great faculty of our nature is infringed upon by disease. The records of medicine are crowded with such instances; indicating a wonderful variety in the kind and degree of these morbid changes; and in some of them a character so strange and unexpected, as to require the full guarantee of evidence which they have actually received. If seeking for a phrase to denote the general nature of such phenomena, that of *dislocation* of memory might best perhaps be employed. But no single term can express the various effects of accident, disease, or decay upon this faculty, so strangely partial in their aspect, and so abrupt in the changes they undergo, that the attempt to classify them is almost as vain as the research into their cause. Those which arise from falls, blows, or other accidents producing concussion, are perhaps the most extraordinary; in the suddenness of their effects, and from the manner in which they disturb and dissever the objects of memory already existing in the mind. Particular passages of life are thus at once obliterated, or the recollection lost of particular classes of facts — the lines of partition in these cases being often such as we could never have recognised but for the changes in question; and suggesting strongly the notion of a separate seat or locality to things thus definitely divided by a mere accident or condition of disease.*

It happens here, as in so many other parts of pathology, that the best understanding of the subject is that drawn from observations of the faculty in its natural state. In memory more especially, the mutual relations of health and disease illustrate what could be known from no other source. Few of its morbid conditions, even those most anomalous, but have some prototype amidst the variations in its natural and healthy exercise. Of all the faculties of mind it is that which permits the greatest diversities, and undergoes the strangest fluctuations. A history might be composed of the differences which mark the memory of different individuals ; and no more curious document could be offered in relation to the intellect of man. It is not the mere distinction of good and bad, or the several grades between them, extraordinary though these diversities are, which would enter into such history. It must record,

---

* These phenomena existing at every time, we may reasonably expect notice of them in the older writers. I select one from Pliny ; an authority of moderate value in most cases, but here the more to be relied upon, from the exact concurrence of the instances he gives, with our own experience. After reciting some remarkable examples of the perfection of memory, he continues ; " Nec aliud est æquè fragile in homine ; morborum, et casûs injurias, atque etiam metus sentiens ; aliàs particulatim, aliàs universa. Ictus lapide, oblitus est literas tantùm. Ex præalto tecto lapsus, matris et adfinium, pro-pinquorumque cepit oblivionem. Alius ægrotus, servorum etiam ; sui verò nominis Messala Corvinus ovator," &c.—*Hist. Nat.* VII.

also, the partial excellences or defaults of memory, as respects its particular objects — the methods by which it is educated and exercised — its relation to the voluntary power of recollection, and to the other intellectual powers — and, finally, its manner of natural decay in old age, as various as' its growth in youth, and yet more remarkable in the analysis it affords of the nature and workings of the faculty.

Nor is this illustration to be drawn from different minds only. We speak, indeed, of the memory of an individual as we are wont to speak of his character, as something single and determinate; — and, in a general sense, there may be reason for so doing. But the daily life of every man presents to close observation, or to his own consciousness, anomalies and inequalities of the faculty, which, if less striking than those of disease, are of the same kind, and illustrate by this resemblance the aberrations of the latter. Under what may be considered the particular condition of memory in each individual, there lie hidden endless diversities and changes — original inequality in its power and readiness, as applied to different objects — the variations it undergoes from the natural incidents of life; and from sleep in particular, the most habitual yet most remarkable of these — the influence upon it of the other faculties, and especially of all the mental emotions, — its varying capacity for improvement at different times of life, and under different modes of exercise — and its dependence on those associations and sequences of thought, from which mainly we derive the recollective power. These, and other conditions which might be named, do all more or less expound the alterations produced by disease;

scarcely one of which is really different in nature, though more anomalous to common observation. Whatever their mystery to our understanding, it is the same which exists as to the operations of memory in its healthy state.

Before proceeding, however, with the discussion, it is well to advert more particularly to the distinction between simple memory, and the act or faculty of recollection, — between the mere assemblage and aggregation of materials in the mind, and the power of recalling and combining them by voluntary effort. This distinction requires to be maintained throughout, since it involves different powers very unequally possessed. Common language, as usual, is vague and indiscriminate on this point; and its phrases cannot be accepted into the argument. Nor do we gain much aid from those metaphysical definitions, which resolve memory altogether into other phenomena of mind, as those of simple and relative suggestion, association, &c.*

* Among modern writers on the subject, Dr. Brown has gone furthest, perhaps, to merge this faculty in other functions and names. The argument of this acute metaphysician leads him even to withdraw recollection from the class of voluntary acts; and to refer it to that of suggestions. The whole discussion is another proof of the dominion which methods and phrases exercise over these abstruse subjects.

In the chapter of Aristotle Περι αναμνησεως, will be found, as I have elsewhere noticed, many valuable remarks upon memory; including the important distinction between simple memory and recollection, between the Μνημονικοι and the Αναμνηστικοι. This great author, as I have elsewhere remarked, deserves a diligent study on all subjects connected with mental physiology. It has been made the reproach, and justly, of the Greek school of philosophy, that while eminent from its attainments in abstract mathematics, its progress in all other branches of knowledge, and especially in the Inductive Sciences, was frustrated by faulty methods of pursuit. The Greek philosophers looked to nature mdeed for certain elementary facts; but their use of

The processes of memory, indeed, are performed by association, and depend on suggestion; but neither of these terms, in their ordinary use, express all that we mean even by simple memory, still less denote the higher power of recollection. It is still but another "contexture of words," with which we are dealing; more convenient, it may be, in some points of application, but not affording us any new or more certain knowledge. For our present purpose we need nothing more than the simple expression of certain assured facts; — viz., that there is a faculty of our mental constitution, by which the successive states of mind passed through, whether of thought or sensation, leave impressions behind of more or less clearness and persistence — that these impressions of former states or acts are dormant to the consciousness, until revived by some new exciting cause — and that such causes are either associations independent of the will; or acts of recollection, in which volition is directly concerned, however we may define its manner of operation.

In this general description of the faculty, the equivocal term is that of *impression*, as denoting the traces of former mental states left behind for future revival.* But in

them was narrowed and perverted by forms of language, rendering their science often one of words rather than of realities. I may refer to some admirable remarks on the subject in Whewell's Philosophy of the Inductive Sciences. To such reproach, however, Aristotle is much less liable than most of the philosophers of his age. He was not merely a diligent collector of facts, but had a right appreciation of them, as the foundation of all true knowledge. The eulogium upon him by Cuvier is the testimony of one illustrious naturalist to the eminent merits of another.

* Some of the more recent results in Photography might almost

truth no single word is competent to express a fact which, familiar though it be, may well justify the perpetual wonder with which it is regarded, not by the unlearned only, but even more by those who have closely studied the phenomena of mind. To explain, indeed, how an image or thought should lie absolutely dormant for years, yet be awakened again after such lapse of time by some chance association of the moment, would be to penetrate into the mystery of our nature far beyond all the attainments of our present, probably of our possible, knowledge. No physical cause that we can assign or surmise approaches even to a solution; and what has hitherto been attempted of this kind is altogether futile in reason and result. The absolute insufficiency of all theory founded on the connexion of memory with organisation, is more strongly felt when we regard those astonishing instances of memory which occasionally occur to our notice — admirable in some

---

tempt one to substitute the term of *image* here; to express the parallel case of an impression made, but wholly hidden from the sense until evolved by other agents. It would be too bold, however, to rest a definition upon such analogy. In the " *Wissenschaft für dic gesammte Heilkunde*, 1836," there is a valuable memoir on the "Phenomena of Memory in the Senses," by Professor Henle; containing some curious notices of the images or outlines which continue, or recur, of objects that have long been intently looked upon. All these analogies are interesting, though they carry us but little in advance of doctrines of a much earlier date. Those who are lovers of Lucretius (and as respects his poetry, who is otherwise?) will recollect the various passages in his Fourth Book, in which he labours to give a sort of material reality to the images of sense and memory. His "Simulacra, Effigiæ, Imagines, Tenues Figuræ," &c., are the efforts of language to endow with substance what we can never know otherwise than in the simple recognition of phenomena.

cases from the universality of the power; in others from its perfection as directed to particular objects, to languages, numbers, persons, or events. What material receptacle can we conceive fitted to contain and conceal these innumerable forms of the past? What material action capable of reviving and recombining them, after years have lapsed away? It is manifest that there is a line of limit here, at which both reason and imagination are arrested; or, if seeking to go beyond it, are lost in error and obscurity.

Yet, while thus incapable of understanding its manner of action, the conviction is forced upon us by the phenomena of memory, that of all the intellectual powers it depends most on organised structure for whatever concerns its completeness, its changes, and decay. We feel it to be ever acting upon materials over the order and distribution of which we have only a partial control. Even when expressly using the powers of recollection, the mind seems almost consciously to be exerting itself on something *without*, which is imperfectly submitted to the will. It courts rather than coerces the instrument, which yet ministers so largely to all its higher functions. In other animals, again, though we cannot prove them to possess the true recollective faculty, we find in many a very extraordinary development of simple memory; frequently more perfect than in man, especially where the functions of the senses are concerned. We have seen how rapidly the faculty is affected in ourselves by disease or physical accidents; and its final decay is antecedent to, and often independent of, that of the higher powers of the understanding.*

---

* In all this we do not affirm that the act of memory is in itself a

The case is hardly less mysterious of things utterly and finally lost to the memory, than of those which are revived at intervals from their latent condition. We must suppose a common physical cause in the two cases, since there is a natural transition from one to the other. Remembrances vivid at first, become progressively feebler with the lapse of time, and in the end disappear. Such, however, are the peculiarities of this faculty, that it is not always easy to determine when the loss is final; for what was seemingly gone for ever may be revived by some new train and association of thought. The surest test probably is, where the reason is assured of certain things having occurred, of which no corresponding trace is found in the recollection. Human life indeed can scarcely be defined without including, as a part of it, what is forgotten together with what is remembered. " The river of Lethe," to use Lord Bacon's words, " runneth as well above ground as below;"—but its fountains, like those of memory, are unseen and inaccessible to our research.

These various phenomena, pertaining to memory in what may be termed its healthy state, are rendered more

---

state or condition of organisation. We merely express what alone we know as probable, that material structure, the excitement and instrument of the mental functions in their relation to the world without, is more closely connected with the operations of memory, than with those of any other faculty.

Though Rochefoucauld intended another and more sarcastic meaning, yet there is a certain truth to our purpose in his maxim:—"Tout le monde se plaint de son memoire, mais personne ne se plaint de son jugement." We feel the memory to be less an integral part of ourselves than the reason.

striking and explicit by accident or disease. We have already stated that there is hardly one morbid incident which is not in part represented in the natural actions of the faculty; but in disease the lines are drawn more strongly, and the changes are more sudden and complete. Those daily or hourly fluctuations in its power, of which every man is conscious to himself, become augmented in degree, are removed more entirely out of the control of the will, and pass into morbid associations of thought and feeling, which disturb and disorder the mind in its every part. If I were writing a treatise on the subject (and it well deserves more ample discussion), it would be desirable not merely to multiply examples to this effect, but to classify the cases recorded, for the clearer understanding of the conclusions they convey. This, however, I cannot here attempt, but must limit myself to such outline as may simply indicate the chief points of inquiry.

The aberrations of memory under the different forms of insanity first require to be noticed; forming, in truth, a large part of the topic before us. For it is difficult to describe any condition to which this name can fitly be applied, without including some change or infirmity of the faculty in question — often blended with its natural workings; but manifested in some error or deficiency of the associations, the consistency and completeness of which are essential to sound reason. The strangeness of many of the facts here observed may well perplex or frustrate all theory. Their combinations and varieties are not fewer than the various forms of madness itself; and in many cases, indeed, it would be impossible to affirm that the defect of memory is not the primary disease, and the aberrations of insanity consequent upon it: such is the difficulty of any just interpretation or definition of these disorders. Instances, however, sometimes occur in which the memory is clear and vivid in particulars, though its results are wholly distorted and misapplied; showing that the faculty may retain its mere mechanical integrity, if such term be allowed, while the higher power to which it ministers is altered and impaired, so as no longer to guide or govern its combinations.

Among the remarkable facts as to memory in cases of insanity, we have to notice the frequent entire forgetfulness, when health of mind is restored, of all that has passed during the period of derangement. This phenomenon is far from uniform, but in many cases sufficiently marked to show that whole periods of time may be swept at once from remembrance; — a circumstance attested also by the effects of certain sudden injuries to the brain, and often very strikingly in the natural decay of old age. Even in the healthy state of the sensorium we have evidence of its much greater aptitude at one period than another to receive and hold firmly the impressions made upon it; so that one class or succession of events may be readily obliterated, while those of an anterior time retain their original force. We have also reason to believe, — and here, again, we derive proof from cases of insanity of periodical kind, — that a recurrence of similar states of the sensorium will often reproduce in certain degree similar trains and associations of memory, which in the cases just named have been wholly absent in the intervals between the attacks. All these phenomena, whether of health or disease, are of great interest in their mutual illustration.

They are subject, as we have already seen, to unceasing variations; but all concur in making it necessary to suppose some organisation, however inconceivable and inscrutable to us in its nature, through which impressions are received and retained; by which they are reproduced at intervals to the mind; and from which they may be finally obliterated by time, accident, or disease.

Among other relations suggested by these curious facts is that between the original force of the impressions received, and their power of resistance to causes of injury or decay. This is a point of great interest, not merely as matter of speculative curiosity, but yet more in its connexion with the practical methods by which the memory may best be educated and maintained. It is certain that the original impressions, subserving to it, are of very various intensity in different persons and at different times. It is certain, also, that there is great variation in each individual as to the facility of receiving, and the vividness of the impressions received, from different objects. The whole art of education, as respects this faculty, consists in regulating the reception of these first impressions, so as to give them firmest hold on the mind; and in furnishing methods by which the power of recollection, in dependence on the will, may best be guided and maintained. But though thus simple in its outline, the education of the memory is in reality rendered a very difficult problem by the numerous natural diversities already mentioned; and one much less capable of being determined by general rules than is commonly believed. There are, however, various points in which its efficiency may be greatly increased by experience and good sense directed toward the result. And these are precisely the instances where physiology and medical knowledge afford suggestions of much value, with reference both to particular cases and to the more general methods employed.

Upon this topic, however, I cannot enter, beyond one remark which bears directly on the subject before us. This is the fact, well attested by experience, that the memory may be seriously, sometimes lastingly injured, by pressing upon it too hardly and continuously in early life. Whatever theory we hold as to this great function of our nature, it is certain that its powers are only gradually developed; and that if forced into premature exercise, they are impaired by the effort. This is a maxim indeed of general import, applying to the condition and culture of every faculty of body and mind; but singularly to the one we are now considering, which forms in one sense the foundation of our intellectual life. A regulated exercise, short of actual fatigue, enlarges its capacity both as to reception and retention; and gives promptitude as well as clearness to its action. But we are bound to refrain from goading it by constant and laborious efforts in early life, and before the instrument has been strengthened to its work, or it decays under our hands. We lose its present power, and often enfeeble it for all future use.

Even where, by technical contrivances, the youthful memory has been crowded with facts and figures, injury is often done thereby to the growth of that higher part of the faculty, which recollects and combines its materials for intellectual purposes. And this is especially true, when the subjects pressed on the mind are those not naturally congenial to it — a distinction very real in itself, and

partially recognised by all, yet often unduly neglected in
our systems of education. The necessity must be admitted
in practice, of adopting certain average rules, under which
the majority of cases may be included. But special
instances are ever before us, where the mind by its constitution is so unfitted for particular objects, that the
attempt to force the memory or other faculties upon them,
is not merely fruitless, but hazardous in result. It is
tersely said by Hippocrates, Φύσεως αντιπραττούσης, κενεα
παντα· — a maxim requiring some qualification, yet never
to be disregarded in our dealings either with the mental or
bodily condition of man.*

Recurring now to the more immediate subject of the influence of disease on the memory, we find, as might have
been expected, that cerebral disorders are those which have
greatest effect. If opinion may be hazarded where absolute proof is so difficult, it would be, that the hemispheres

---

* We find in Quintilian, a writer ever of sound and enlightened
judgment, many valuable precepts as to the cultivation of memory ;
and an earnest reprehension of attempts at a premature development
of this or other faculties. The phrase he applies to such precocious
growths, "Inanibus aristis ante messem flavescunt," has its exact
counterpart in Lord Bacon's description of "that over early ripeness
in years which fadeth betimes."

In the course of my practice I have seen some striking and melancholy instances of the exhaustion of the youthful mind by this over-
exercise of its faculties. In two of these, unattended with paralytic
affection, or other obvious bodily disorder than a certain sluggishness
in the natural functions, the torpor of mind approached almost to
imbecility. Yet here there had before been acute intellect, with
great sensibility ; but these qualities forced by emulation into excess
of exercise, without due intervals of respite, and with habitual deficiency of sleep. Of the importance of the latter point I have spoken
in a preceding chapter.

of the brain are the portions of structure most closely connected with this function; both as respects the impressions
received, and the associations and suggestions which serve
to the recollective power. Various reasons, direct and
indirect, might be alleged in support of this view; some
of which will be noticed in a succeeding chapter. A main
reason is the fact, that any obvious changes in this part of
the brain are always attended with some alteration in the
memory. That change which is denoted, (somewhat
loosely perhaps) by the term of *softening,* furnishes many
striking instances of it. A certain vague wandering of
the recollection often occurs as the first indication of the
disease; while its progress is attended by increasing incapacity, either for receiving new impressions, or recalling
and combining those of earlier date.

Under all conditions of pressure on the brain, however
produced, we witness similar effects of disturbance; modified in kind and degree by the amouut of pressure, the time
of its duration, and probably by other less obvious causes.*
Partial and singular lapses of memory, recurring irre-
gularly, are often noticed a short time before an apoplectic
attack, or other cerebral seizure; and may usually be received as warning of their approach. When more continuous pressure has come on, the gradations of change
may be traced, from the slight confusion or stupor, hardly
to be distinguished from sleep, into that complete comatose
state, in which all the faculties are suspended to outward
observation, whatever their condition within.

---

* On all that relates to pressure on the brain, the reader may well
be advised to consult Dr. Borrows's excellent treatise on this subject.

It is certain, however, that disturbance to the memory may arise from too feeble, as well as from over-excited circulation through the brain. This we might be prepared to expect from general analogy; but it is proved to us also in various cases of bodily disorder. We have evidence of still more familiar kind in the common occurrences of life. The powers of recollection and thought become confused or lost either from violent action or excessive fatigue. No man can think or remember clearly while running rapidly; nor can any one go through a laborious recollection when the body is exhausted and feeble. I have often known memory, thus transiently failing from fatigue or the debility of disease, restored by the stimulus of a moderate quantity of wine; and so suddenly as to show that the want of due excitement to the circulation was the cause of the failure.* But besides this passing effect of momentary exhaustion, there are more chronic states of similar kind, where the memory is enfeebled for considerable periods of time, without being permanently affected. Though there is difficulty in defining this result, from the fluctuations the faculty is ever undergoing, yet common observation, as well as medical experience, attests the reality of the fact.

---

* I find in my notes a curious example in my own case of this transient failure of memory from bodily fatigue. I descended on the same day two very deep mines in the Hartz mountains, remaining some hours underground in each. While in the second mine, and exhausted both from fatigue and inanition, I felt the utter impossibility of talking longer with the German Inspector who accompanied me. Every German word and phrase deserted my recollection; and it was not until I had taken food and wine, and been some time at rest, that I regained them again.

The effects of paralytic disorders upon the memory are much more striking from their permanence, and the singular character they assume.   It is here especially that we perceive that strange forgetfulness and misplacement of language, of which I have given a few instances in the early part of this chapter, — cases where the ideas still remaining distinct, words are partially wanting for their expression; or others, by an inexplicable perversion, are substituted, having no relation to the intended sense.   I might largely multiply such examples from my notes or from other sources, were this necessary.   It is an interesting question whether there is any form of paralysis, more than another, concerned in this particular effect ?   I have sought for evidence on the subject, but without acquiring any that is satisfactory ; — if ever obtained, it must be from a larger average of cases, than can probably come within the scope of private practice.   It somewhat facilitates the examination of these results, though not lessening their singularity, to regard them as residual effects of the original paralytic seizure.   As in the case with the voluntary organs after such attack, the first loss of power is the most complete ; its restoration very gradual, and involving those inequalities, particularly in the recollection of language, which are so curiously testified in the cases referred to.*   After passing through different stages of recovery, the

---

* In speaking of the first loss of voluntary power in paralysis as being most complete, I must make exception for the curious fact, that the palsied state often goes on increasing for a day or two after the attack, when it reaches a maximum point, from which recovery of power begins. A probable reason might be assigned for this ; but the discussion would be out of place here.

M

memory does now and then regain in the end its former state; though the instances are far more frequent, where the faculty remains imperfect, or is further injured by the occurrence of fresh paralytic attacks.

The causes and course of epilepsy are so various, that it is difficult to determine the exact nature and amount of its effects. It is certain, however, that every epileptic seizure not merely disturbs the memory at the moment, but for some time afterwards, in degree proportionate to its severity; and that the frequent repetition of these attacks permanently impairs it. The periodical tendency also of this remarkable disease frequently shows itself in the effects thus produced on the mental faculties. Where the intervals between the fits are long and somewhat regular, we often notice a disturbance of mind, gradually augmenting until the moment of the attack; and subsiding again into the ordinary state, after its immediate effects have passed away. It is one of the many indications afforded by this disease, of a cause of irritation gradually accumulating in the system, and *discharged*, as we may best describe it, by the epileptic fit.*

It may be affirmed as a general fact that the memory is affected, more or less, by every febrile state of the body,—whether through primary effect on the brain, or indirectly by changes in the cerebral circulation, it is not easy to determine. The latter view, perhaps, is the more probable; inasmuch as the recollection, sluggish and inert in its operations during the cold stage of fever, becomes often morbidly active and vivid in the hot stage following.

* See Chap. XXII. of Medical Notes and Reflections, "On Morbid Actions of Intermittent kind."

This difference of condition accords with what we observe in slighter degree where no disease is present. The memory, as we have seen, has its natural variations of action, equally with every other function of mind and body. It may become inert or confused from simple exhaustion; or vigorous and acute from repaired power and fresh excitement. These changes, in truth, are closely connected with the causes which produce the alternations of sleep and waking, and may almost be regarded as an expression of the same phenomena.

During the severe Epidemic Influenzas (as they have been conventionally called) of late years, I have very often noticed a distinct influence on the memory of patients affected with the disorder, even in its earliest stage — a fact further attested by their own consciousness and expressions. Whatever the material causes of this singular malady, they are clearly of sedative kind, producing much general prostration of the vital and mental powers. The functions of memory show this adynamic state by a sort of torpor and inability, approaching to the condition we so often observe in typhoid fever; and expressing, in fact, the same type of disorder; an inference confirmed by many other evidences in the history of this epidemic.

The natural decay of memory in old age, though not in any obvious proportion to the decline of those powers which connect us more directly with the external world, must be admitted as a fact in our mental constitution. It depends, doubtless, on those gradual changes in the brain, whatsoever their nature, which in other cases are anticipated by accident or disease. Where there has been no express disorder of this organ, and where the faculty was originally strong, it is occasionally preserved to a very late period of existence, and amidst much of general decay. Instances to this effect, some of them very remarkable, will be familiar to every one. But even in these exceptional cases we rarely fail to note, as time goes on, some partial deficiency in the memory of names or words, or things of recent occurrence; and a more lengthened and laborious effort in every act of recollection. These are generally, indeed, the earliest tokens of change in the faculty; and if no more urgent disease intervene, the further alteration is in general merely a gradual increase of such enfeeblement. Where the case is otherwise, and the changes more rapid, they still resemble in great part those resulting from disease at an earlier time of life; or even yet more, the common condition of dreaming. The memory becomes vague and incoherent in its associations — the power of combining and directing them by will is greatly impaired — the trains of recollection are abruptly broken by the slightest incident or suggestion — the events of whole periods of life are often forgotten, while those more remote in time are brought into transient remembrance — names, words, and numbers are lost, or come before the mind only to beget confusion.

This is the memory in the extreme decay of age, when life approaches in reality to the state of a dream, and may best be so represented. In a chapter of my former work (On the Medical Treatment of Old Age) I have spoken on this subject, and given some instances illustrative of it.*

* " In a lady of ninety-one, whom I am now attending, the decay of the mind shows itself especially in the dependence of the course of ideas on the sound of words. A word, or even part of a word, of

The discussion is one of great interest in many ways. We obtain from it various evidence that the enfeeblement of the several faculties is not in the same ratio as to time; and that, in regard to memory, the losses are not equal of the ideas of different classes, and different periods of acquisition. Whether from diversity of state in the recipient organs; the frequency of intermediate revival to the mind; or from other causes, it seems certain that the incidents and impressions of earlier life are better preserved than those of recent occurrence.

The capacity for receiving and fixing new impressions appears, indeed, to decline sooner than the power of recalling and using those formerly received; and even when this power ceases with advancing age, these images of a former time still frequently steal upon the mind, and strangely blend themselves with the incidents of the passing moment. Again, we find reason to believe, as respects the decay of memory, that the ability to recollect words and names is lost earlier and more readily than that of events, whether in effect of old age or disease. It is difficult to obtain assurance on these several points, where the diversity is so great in different cases, and the evidence so precarious in all. But I mention them as curious subjects of inquiry,

double application, will suddenly, and without the consciousness of change, carry off the mind to a new and wholly foreign subject. In another elderly patient, whose memory is singularly tenacious as to persons and detached events of past life, there is a singular incapacity of associating them together by any reasonable link; and the slightest relations of time or place suffice to carry the mind wholly astray from its subject. Such instances, by no means uncommon, have close kindred to the state of dreaming; the power of regulating the course of thought being similarly impaired in both cases."

and doubtless admitting of more certain results from
further examination.

I must not close this chapter without adverting to a
question which often comes before the medical man —
suggested by his own thoughts or the anxiety of others —
whether any thing can be done to restore and repair the
memory thus injured by disease or gradual decay? The
candid physician will not pretend to more than indirect
methods of attaining this object. We have no immediate
access by medicines or specific remedies to this great
faculty of our nature. It is true that there are many
physical agents capable of affecting the memory, through
their influence on the brain; but by far the greater
number, if not all of these, act by disturbing the function,
and we hold none in our hands which are capable in
any direct manner of restoring its integrity.

Nevertheless, the office of the physician is far from
being a negative one in this matter. The removal or
abatement of injurious causes affecting the brain, does
often restore its efficiency to the memory thus impaired;
nor is the benefit rendered equivocal by its being obtained indirectly, and as a secondary object, and with
little cognisance of the relation of means to the end.
Such indirect methods, and the same ignorance of proximate relations, pervade every part of medical practice,
without lessening the efficacy of the results drawn from a
sound experience. Each case, then, according to this
view, must furnish suggestions from its particular symptoms; the general principle being, that whatever tends to
produce a healthy state of brain, in all its functions, best

contributes to repair default in the memory or recollective power. Whether undue pressure be concerned; or a cerebral circulation too violent or too feeble; or concussion; or other more obscure injury to the nervous substance, equally must this principle form the foundation of all that can be rightly attempted in medical treatment.

Its admission renders it needless to dilate on this part of the subject. If the injury to the faculty is from any sudden cause,—as paralysis, or bodily accident, or mental shock—time, quiet, and the removal of obvious causes of disturbance, comprise all that can be done, in addition to the ordinary medical treatment of such cases. The same as to epilepsy. The heavy sleep or stupor following the fit should never be interrupted by attempts, worse than useless, to excite the faculties into action. This state itself provides naturally for their best and most speedy restoration. In all such csses premature exercises of the memory, testified to be so by the labour and difficulty attending them, should be sedulously prevented. They seriously disturb the brain, and retard the return of the function to its natural state.

For the relief of the effects produced by febrile diseases, or other causes of exhaustion of the nervous energy, the same principle must be applied. The memory returns as the disease abates, or as the strength is restored; and nothing can be done more directly to accelerate its restoration. In such cases, indeed, we are seldom called upon to attempt it.

This demand is more frequently made where the faculty is impaired from slower changes in the brain, and notably from the decay of old age. Here no obvious cause is present; and the patient himself, or those around him, conscious of the change, naturally seek to know whether any thing can be effected to obviate or retard it. I have already said how little ought to be attempted in such cases beyond what may conduce to the general health. The only other means the physician can rightly suggest are negative in kind—such as may guard the faculty from the ill-judged management of patients themselves. Its progressive decay cannot be prevented; but, to a certain extent, it may be husbanded by care and temperate use. The first mistrust of memory leads many persons to tax it in the way of trial, and through a vague notion of improvement. They persist in harrassing efforts to recover a word, a name, or a number, under the feeling that discomfiture is a declaration of inability;—whereas the labour of the attempt is in itself the cause of present failure; and of future mischief, if often repeated. Even in the full vigour of life there is a natural limit to the use of that power by which the mind thus concentrates itself in inward examination of its own operations. This limit is much more closely drawn in old age. The sense of fatigue or confusion coming upon the faculties from the effort is the certain test of its unfitness; and the advice should be in every such case to abandon the attempt at once, and engage the mind on other topics. This is not always easy of accomplishment, especially when the will has become infirm of purpose and power. But the principle is clear, and must ever be kept in view.

We often find the suspicion of failure of memory occurring earlier in life; oftenest, perhaps, in those in whom the faculty is most powerful, and who are proportionally jealous as to any tokens of decay. It is here, as with respect to the exercise of the voluntary organs; the apprehension of inability actually creates it; and one failure begets another. The experience of every man's life furnishes examples of this; the explanation being that which I have given in a preceding chapter. The mind cannot be simultaneously in two states of thought; and the anxious doubt of success interrupts by its presence those trains of association upon which recollection depends. Restored confidence in such cases repairs the failure, by excluding this cause of disturbance, and enabling the mind to concentrate itself again upon its object.*

Much more might be written on the various phenomena — familiar as a part of our constitution, but more wonderful to our reason — which form the subject of this chapter. The plan of the present volume, however, limits me on this topic, as on others, to such outline as may suffice to indicate the actual state of our knowledge regarding it, and the questions which we must consider still open to future inquiry.

* Many curious instances might be given to illustrate this need of disengagement of the mind in recollection. In reciting a passage of poetry from memory, there is generally better success from trusting to the mere mechanism of the faculty, than from any effort to guide it by thought or suggestion. A line, laboriously and vainly sought for, will often flash upon the mind, when the search has been discontinued.

Sir Philip Warwick, in his Memoirs, says of Lord Strafford, "His memory was great, and he made it greater by confiding in it." Quintilian expresses, in another form, the practical value of this confidence, in relation to the business of life. "Memoriæ plerumque inhæret fidelius, quod nullâ scribendi securitate laxatur."

CHAP. VIII.

ON THE BRAIN AS A DOUBLE ORGAN.

I AM not sure that this subject of the relation of the two hemispheres of the brain has yet been followed into all the consequences which may, more or less directly, result from it. Symmetry of arrangement on the two sides of the body is common indeed to all the organs of animal life.* But the *doubleness* of the brain, like all besides pertaining to this great nervous centre, offers much more of curious speculation than the same constitution of other parts. That unity of consciousness in perception, volition, memory, thought, and passion, which characterises the mind in its healthy state (" illud quod sentit, quod sapit, quod vult, quod viget"), is singularly contrasted with the division into two equal portions, of the material organ which more immediately ministers to these high functions. Yet, on the other hand, in the almost exact symmetry of form and composition of each hemisphere — in their relation precisely similar to the organs of sense and voluntary motion on each side the body — and in the structure of the

* The distinction established by modern physiologists between the animal and vital organs, as respects the symmetry of the sides, is an important one, and well sanctioned by facts. The symmetry presented to us in the former, is one example of that more general law or tendency to such arrangement, which we find, under different forms, so largely prevailing both in the organic and inorganic parts of nature.

nervous connexions subsisting between them, we find argument, not merely for the correspondence of functions, but even for that unity or individuality, of which consciousness is the interpreter to all. This unity, indeed, actually exists; and is therefore of necessity compatible with the conformation of the brain as a double organ, even had we no such presumption to refer to.*

Here, it must be admitted, we are close upon that line, hardly to be defined by the human understanding, which separates material organisation and actions from the proper attributes of mind — the structure which ministers to perception from the percipient — the instruments of voluntary power from the will itself. Our existence may be said to lie on each side this boundary; yet with a chasm between, so profound and obscure, that, though perpetually traversing it in all the functions of life, we have no eye to penetrate its depths. If we sometimes seem to obtain a show of further discovery (and human thought has exhausted itself in the effort), this arises generally from the deception of language, which gives the appearance of advancing, when in truth we are but treading in our former steps.

* Though the nervous system in all its parts, with the exception of that belonging to the great sympathetic, is subject to fewer anomalies than any other organs of the body, yet are these deviations more frequent in man than in many of the mammalia most nearly approaching to him in structure; an observation made originally by Vic d'Azyr, and confirmed by later physiologists. It is further to be noticed, as an anatomical fact, that in the brain and spinal marrow, the external parts on the two sides are less exactly symmetrical than those within; the surface of the brain showing this perhaps more distinctly than any other part. See Meckel's *Handbuch der Menschlichen Anatomie*, vol. i. ch. 3.

While approaching these limits, however, in the subject before us, it may be pursued to a certain extent within the boundary. Many of the questions of greatest interest here have not more concern with materialism, than have the facts which connect dreaming and intoxication with certain physical changes occurring in the body. The intellectual existence, of which consciousness and personal identity are the simplest expressions, but which spreads itself out into the endless varieties of thought and feeling (μη χωριστη κατα μεγεθος αλλα κατα λογον), has been given us, subject to external agents from the first moment of life; both in the functions of health, and under the various circumstances of disease.* And any results we

---

* I know no happier expression of personal identity, and its relation to the nature of mind, than that of Mr. J. Smith of Cambridge. " Mere matter could never thus stretch forth its feeble force, and spread itself over all its own former pre-existences." The same argument (for the force of the remark renders it such) may be followed into the future, as well as fetched from the past; and still more remarkably, as respects the intellectual existence of man. By facts already attained, and methods of thought previously acquired, the mind becomes capable of passing beyond its actual knowledge, and gaining what may be deemed certainty as to the result of combinations which have never yet existed; or, if existing, have never before been the subject of human observation. Physical science abounds in examples, where predictions thus made have been verified in the event. The conversion, by two reflections in glass, of the plane polarization of light into the circular, is an instance of the highest class of such generalizations directed towards the future, and realised in the progress of research. The undulatory doctrine of light offers other examples no less remarkable, in the anticipation by a profound theory, of complex effects, wholly unknown as facts, and even in seeming contradiction to all analogies of the science; yet which experiment has since established as real, and in harmony with the other laws of light. The loftiest attributes and objects of a

may obtain from the inquiry are but further examples of this essential condition of our being.

If making a single comment here upon the question of materialism, it would be that the advocate for an immaterial principle is often unjust to his argument, in his assiduity to rid himself of those facts which attest the close and constant action of matter upon mind. They are too palpable, not merely in matters of sense, but also as regards the purely mental processes, to admit of any evasion. His true doctrine lies beyond this, in asserting a principle submitted indeed to these influences, but different from them; — capable of independent changes and actions within itself; — and, above all, capable of self-

philosophical spirit all lie in this direction. Here it is, in passing from "the region of facts to that of laws," that man takes his peculiar position in the scale of created beings; and here, also, that the intellect of one man stretches furthest beyond that of another.

Under the same aspect (for all the higher views in science associate themselves into principles of common truth) we may best view the great argument regarding causation — the "selva oscura" of philosophy, as it has been ever rendered by the inefficiency or ambiguity of language applied to the subject. The frequent misuse of the term *final causes* (perhaps even the adoption of the phrase at all) may be cited as one of the chief sources of error. No proof of efficient and intelligent causation, as distinguished from the bare sequence of events, is more complete and convincing than the power we possess of predicting results which have never occurred to us before, but which arise out of laws so fixed and general, that we can safely anticipate the unknown from what we already know. In pursuing science along this path (the happiest exercise of man's divination), we obtain certainty of an intelligent cause from a source hardly separable from the consciousness of our own intellectual existence. And in thus making the highest efforts of the human faculty the interpreters of the principle of divine causation, we bring our conception of moral cause into closest relation with the physical, and acquire not only elevation, but distinctness and stability in all our views on the subject.

regulation in those functions of thought and feeling, to which external agents minister in the various processes of life. The ministering agents may become disturbing ones, and such they frequently are to a singular extent; but in this we have no proof of identity. Whatever of reason we can apply to an argument insuperable by human reason, is against it. And the record of such instances is wholly comprised within that one great relation, which pervades every part of our present being; but the intimate nature of which is a sealed book to human research.*

We may then as fairly reason upon the states or changes of mind depending on the brain as a double organ, as we do on the effects of palpable injury or disease affecting it directly or indirectly through other parts of the nervous system. And, indeed, in the doubleness of the nerves and other organs of animal life we obtain a series of phenomena which variously interpret these more obscure disturbances in the mental faculties; and make it probable that some, at least, depend on changes in the relation of parts, to which a strict unity of action belongs in the healthy state.

Paralytic affections, whether of the organs of sense or vo-

---

* It is an old argument, but one so pertinent as well to bear repetition, that we know as much of, and can as clearly prove, the separate existence of mind, as of matter. Cuvier strongly expresses this : — " Le matérialisme est un hypothèse, d'autant plus hazardé, que la philosophie ne peut donner aucune preuve directe de l'existence effective de la matière."—*Regne Animale.*

Without quoting it as an argument, there is pleasure in recurring to the noble language of Plato, when treating of the soul of man.

Σκοπεῖ δὴ...τῷ μὲν θείῳ καὶ ἀθανάτῳ, καὶ νοητῷ, καὶ μονοειδεῖ, καὶ ἀδιαλύτῳ, καὶ ἀεὶ ὡσαύτως καὶ κατὰ ταῦτα ἔχοντι ἑαυτῷ ὁμοιότατον εἶναι ψυχήν.   And again, Αὐτὸ, κατ᾽ αὐτὸ, μετ᾽ αὐτὸ, μονειδὲς ἀεὶ ὄν.

luntary motion, are the most distinct and familiar examples
of morbid results connected with this doubleness of structure.   However numerous the facts now collected, there
is still much to be learnt as to these affections; and particularly regarding the parts of the brain or spinal marrow
with which they are severally associated, and the nature
of the diseased changes on which they depend.   Modern
anatomy has, with much reason and great success, been
directed especially to those portions of the nervous system
which form, by decussation, the commissures or bonds of
union between the cerebral hemispheres, as well as to those
which seem to connect the sentient and motor nerves in
their course and functions.   These are manifestly parts of
singular importance to the whole animal economy.   On
the connexions afforded by the Corpus Callosum and the
other commissures depend, it may be presumed, the unity
and completeness of the functions of this double organization, as well as the translation of morbid actions from one
side to the other.   And any breach in the integrity of the
union, and of the relations thus established, may tend no
less than disease in the respective parts themselves, to
disturb the various actions of the brain and nervous
system.

It is true that the observations made, through experiments or accidental lesions of the commissures, give
results quite as equivocal as those on other portions of the
brain — or even more obscure, from the difficulty of reaching these parts without such structural injury as greatly
to impair the evidence.   The observations of Reil, Rolando,
and other physiologists, though valuable, cannot be considered as leading to any assured conclusions.   Still it is

probable, or even certain, that many phenomena of sensorial disorder have their origin in these connecting parts
especially, as the seat of disease; and some cases of idiotcy
are recorded in which examination after death showed their
deficiency or disorganization. The decussating fasciculi
of the anterior pyramid are a portion of such structure,
where any morbid cause might be likely to produce peculiar effects; and to which, in fact, we must look for one of
the most remarkable conditions in hemiplegia, viz. the
relation of the seat of injury in the brain to the side of the
body in which paralysis occurs. The connexion of the
two eyes in natural vision and under disease, offer some
curious evidences on this subject; and here the facts are
more distinct in certain other animals, (as birds for example,) than in man. But it is probable that minute
anatomy — aided, as it now so largely is, by pathology —
may hereafter furnish us with many more proofs to this
effect than we at present possess.*

---

* We have reason, as is well known, to attribute to some morbid
cause, affecting for a time the commissure of the optic nerves where
the semi-decussation occurs, the singular phenomenon of *Suffusio
dimidians*, or *Hemiopia*, where one half only of the field of vision is
perceived by the mind. That the interruption causing this deficiency
takes place here, is made more probable by its being usually a transient occurrence. I have known a patient, suffering under various
symptoms of diseased brain, who frequently saw only half his face
when looking into a glass. Very recently I have met with an instance where a father and daughter had each the liability to this
affection. These cases are by no means infrequent; and in almost
every one, I have noticed that the occurrence of the attack was
followed by intense head-ache.

The remarkable case of Dr. Wollaston is known from his own
description, and was too well explained by the circumstances of

Without actual paralysis, however, or any obvious default of the external organs, there is a frequent dissimilarity or inequality of the two sides of the body as regards their nervous condition; testified by differences in sensibility and voluntary power; and also, though more ambiguously, by liability to morbid affections, connected with some of the proper functions of organic life. The observation of such inequality, whether congenital or proceeding from changes in the progress of life, is often made by patients themselves. I have known a case where

cerebral disease, which closed the days of this extraordinary and excellent man. During the latter period of his life, when the existence of such disease, and the certainty of its event, were alike known to him, he was accustomed to take exact note of the changes progressively occurring in his sensations, memory, and voluntary power. He made daily experiments to ascertain their amount, and described the results in a manner which can never be forgotten by those who heard him. It was a mind unimpaired in its higher parts, watching over the physical phenomena of approaching death; and, what well deserves note, watching over the progressive change in those functions which seem nearest to the line separating material from intellectual existence.

In a paper by Professor Alison, " On single and correct vision, by double and inverted images on the retina" (*Trans. of Royal Society of Edinburgh*, vol. xiii.), will be found some striking and original views on this curious subject. And we have since obtained a very remarkable addition to our knowledge of the phenomena of vision, and the relation of the two images to the actual perceptions of the mind, from the researches of Professor Wheatstone; whose beautiful instrument, the Stereoscope—with the more recent illustration derived from his Pseudoscope — have furnished experimental demonstration bearing upon the most difficult parts of this theory. Sir David Brewster, to whom science is so deeply indebted in every part, has further elucidated the mechanism of vision from double images by an apparatus, so contrived as to imitate the relative condition of the two eyes, in receiving and transmitting impressions from without.

N

blisters, and all other external stimulants, acted more powerfully on one side of the body than the other. Andral mentions an instance where perspiration occurred only on one side of the body; and I myself have seen a singular example of such limitation to one half the face; with the peculiarity, however, of this perspiration being morbid in kind and degree.* I may mention, as another instance (more singular from a tube being concerned), certain inflammations of the larynx and trachea, in which the vascular injection is found to be limited to one half the tube, the other half preserving the ordinary appearance. It is stated by the eminent pathologist just named, that he has made this observation in several cases where one lung only was disordered, and this always on the same side as the affection of the trachea.

Hemicrania is one of the most familiar forms of headache, and it is well known with what exactness the pain often follows the median line. I have recently seen a case where, in hemicranial headaches, coming on generally every fortnight, there has occurred for some months past a regular alternation of the sides affected; so that the patient has got into the habit of reckoning with assurance which side will next suffer. It has been observed that deafness

---

* The patient here was a gentleman about thirty-six years of age, and of good health; save that, on the slightest exertion of speaking, eating, or emotion of mind, sweat broke out profusely in drops from the right side of the face, strictly defined by the median line, the other side remaining in its natural state. The complaint had existed four or five years, coming on without obvious cause. An instance is mentioned to me, by a medical friend, of a horse that sweated only on one side of the body; having also liability to giddiness, when heated, which made it dangerous to use him.

is more frequent in the left ear; but this, if it be true, depends probably on some external cause.

It is needless, however, to multiply instances which are so common in practice, and which do not contradict, but rather illustrate by exception, those still more numerous cases where a distinct symmetry is observed in morbid affections of the two sides.* Both conditions are easily and equally explicable on the simple view that, together with *similarity*, there is *separation* to a great extent, of the structure and actions of the two halves of the body. We find bilateral symmetry, with few exceptions, of the cerebral and spinal systems, of the muscles of voluntary motion, of the blood vessels therewith connected. But the division is a fact of the same importance as the doubleness, and guides us to conclusions of equal interest. Pathology, as we have stated, undoubtedly sanctions the general view that where organs are symmetrical as respects the median line of the body—or even where they contain a median line in their own structure, — there is a frequent tendency in morbid actions to terminate at these lines. It might be worth while, as a part of pathological history, to collect and class the various cases of this description, with an

---

* On this subject of the Symmetry of Disease, there are two interesting papers, by Dr. William Budd and Mr. Paget, in vol. xxv. of the Med. Chirurgical Transactions. Now that we are able to recognise so many causes of disease in morbid states of the blood — one of the greatest steps of advancement in modern medical science — it is easy to conceive how these changes in the circulating fluid, acting on parts exactly similar in texture and function, should produce corresponding morbid effects on the two sides of the body.

ulterior view to the suggestions they may afford to medical treatment. *

In the examples we have already given, there is
sufficient proof of the frequent difference of the two sides
as to the numerous conditions of sensibility, — this disparity depending occasionally, it may be, on the external
organs serving to sensation, or on the nerves which associate these organs with the sensorium; but sometimes connected, we have reason to believe, with inequality in those
corresponding parts of the brain which more directly
minister to the perceptions of the mind.   The effects of
injury or disease furnish various proofs of the latter fact;
though the same result may conceivably also occur as a
consequence of some congenital dissimilarity in the two
hemispheres.

Differences in the voluntary power of the two sides are so
far subordinate to the disparity of power and use in the
two arms, that it is difficult often to appreciate the influence of other causes, unless when they reach the extent of
actual disease.   Whence this disparity itself proceeds, and
how it acquires such uniformity, are points still uncertain.
That some organic difference is concerned may be inferred
from the exceptions to the habit being occasionally con-

---

* In pursuing this inquiry, regard must be had to the doctrine
now held by some of the best anatomists, that all the organs of the
body are symmetrically double in their earliest state; even those
which subsequently form cavities or continuous tubes. This part
of pathology is altogether a very interesting one; and the tendency
described above, though often hidden or obscured by other circumstances, yet is sufficiently certain to form a principle of frequent
application in the treatment of disease.

genital, and frequent in the same family. Were it not for this fact (which is, however, of rare occurrence), the view given in the subjoined note might, perhaps, be received as a probable one.* It is affirmed by Meckel, that a great majority of cases of mal-conformation occur on the left side of the body; and, as far as my own observation goes, the remark is well founded. Whether it be so or not, the frequent difference in the two sides, as respects liability to morbid actions and sensations, cannot be denied; and the observations already made show in how many instances there is reason to attribute to variations in the two sides of the brain; or, perhaps also, to some diversity in that part of the system of the spinal cord most directly associated with the sensorial functions.† In-

* The inquiry as to the physical cause of this difference has a sort of local limitation in the fact that there is no corresponding difference in the lower limbs. May we not find explanation in the position of the heart on the left side of the body? In actions requiring the use of only one arm, a very slight circumstance might determine the preference; and such circumstance would be found in the difficulty or hindrance to the heart's action, created by certain positions and motions of the left arm. If this be insufficient to explain the degree of uniformity, must we not look further, to the tendency all habits have to become hereditary in a long series of generations?

In the remarkable researches of M. Dubois Reimond, on the evolution of electricity by muscular contraction, he found a greater deflection of the needle by the forcible contractions of the muscles of the right arm than by those of the left. This result, however, might have been expected, whatever the view taken as to the precise relation of the phenomena.

† Or, looking to the reflex nervous function as distinct from the true cerebral, and depending on an especial organisation in the system of the spinal cord, disparity of the two sides may equally exist here; and influence the actions, both in health and disease, which depend on this function.

dependently of other organic causes, one side of the brain
has been occasionally found more affected with atrophy
than the other, and this cannot exist without showing
itself in some corresponding inequality throughout every
part of the body.

Bichat is the author who has dwelt most explicitly on
the symmetry in the organs of animal life, and the effects
of default in this, either from natural conformation or
disease. The relation of the symmetry of double parts to
unity of action and individuality of result, is so important
in all the economy of life, that every deviation from it
deserves careful notice; and especially where it is associated with some definite disease of the nervous system.
Hitherto I have spoken principally of the effects of such
disparity upon the senses and voluntary power; but must
we not look to the functions of memory and association
also, as probably affected in various ways by unequal or
incongruous action in the two hemispheres of the brain?
These faculties (if indeed we can rightly define them as
separate) obviously depend for their operation on organised
structure; and, as we have shown in the last chapter, are
only partially subject to the intellect and will. Their
unity of action is as needful as that of the senses and
voluntary powers, and may be presumed as closely connected with symmetry of the two cerebral hemispheres;
admitting, what cannot be denied, that each hemisphere
partakes in the organisation required for these functions.
Without referring, then, to those more striking consequences of accident or disease, where the memory and
associations are suddenly altered or impaired, we must
admit the likelihood of analogous effects from slower,

slighter, or more transient deviations from equality. It is difficult to conceive any such deviation to exist without the occurrence of some change, however this may be obscured to our observation.

A theory has been adopted by some, in relation to the mental faculties, that each side of the brain is separately capable of fulfilling the functions, whatever they be, in which this organ ministers to them. And this view has been applied, although somewhat vaguely, to explain the alleged fact that every portion of the brain has been found in different cases the subject of disease, without obvious disturbance of the faculties of the mind.* Though the evidence here is insufficient for the whole fact assumed, yet it is doubtless true to a very considerable extent, and the conclusion thence derived is not without plausibility. But were we to admit the assumption that a given portion of one hemisphere could minister to a certain function in all its completeness, the action being suspended of the corresponding part on the opposite side, yet is there no proof that such substitution can immediately take place; and still less any presumption that it is likely to occur where the functions of the affected part are not suspended, but merely altered and deranged. The distinction in the latter case is manifest; and it is only partially obviated by

---

* Among the more remarkable cases to this effect is that recorded by Cruveilhier; where one hemisphere, throughout every part, was reduced by atrophy to half the dimensions of the other, yet with retention of all the mental faculties. The latter statement is obviously the doubtful part of this case; as will be well understood by all who are accustomed carefully to look into the evidence belonging to such points.

referring to those phenomena of sensation where the organ
of one side appears under certain circumstances to perform
all that belongs to the entire function.   The instances are
as frequent of disturbance to the common action of both,
from morbid changes in which one alone is originally
concerned.

Still there is one important fact here, which seems to be
attested by as much evidence as the subject admits of.
In every instance where there exists any corresponding
lesion or disease on each side of the brain, there we are
sure to find some express injury or impairment of the mental
functions; and generally permanent, whatever be its particular nature.   The bearing of this fact is obvious, even
though we cannot follow it into those details which might
render it conclusive as to the particular relations of the two
hemispheres.

The considerations already stated bring us immediately
to the question, whether some of the aberrations of mind,
which come under the name of insanity, are not due to
incongruous action of this double structure, to which perfect unity of action belongs in the healthy state?   When
the functions which directly place us in relation to the
world without, are liable to so much disorder from this
source, it is easy to conceive that the intellectual part also
may suffer change: the result either of disturbed perceptions, of irregular associations, or of some unequal consciousness or exercise of voluntary power.   The subject is
very obscure, and all proof difficult of attainment; but I
think it more probable than otherwise that such inequality
is the cause of some among the many forms of mental
derangement.   Obvious lesion or active disease are con-

cerned in numerous cases; and these, when affecting one
side of the brain only, may produce their results by disturbing the proper correspondence, or unity of action, of
the two sides.   But there are presumably other cases
where, without manifest injury of structure, there may be
inequality enough in the actions of the two hemispheres
respectively, to disorder and derange the trains of thought,
for longer or shorter time, and in every variety of change
and degree.   The actual number and diversity of such
mental phenomena, both in health and disease, may well
warrant us in seeking explanation from any source, not
incompatible with the laws of organised life.

It has been a familiar remark that in certain states of
mental derangement, as well as in some cases of hysteria
which border closely upon it, there appear, as it were, two
minds; one tending to correct by more just perceptions,
feelings, and volitions, the aberrations of the other; and
the relative power of these influences varying at different
times.   Cases of this singular kind cannot fail to be in
the recollection of every medical man.   I have myself seen
many such, in which there occurred great disorder of mind
from this sort of double-dealing with itself.   In some
cases there would seem to be a double series of sensations;
the real and unreal objects of sense impressing the individual so far simultaneously that the judgment and acts of
mind are disordered by their concurrence.   In other instances the incongruity is chiefly marked in the moral
feelings,—an opposition far more striking than that of
incongruous perceptions, and forming one of the most
painful studies to the observer of mental disease.   We
have often occasion to witness acts of personal violence

committed by those who have at the very time a keen
sense of the wrong, and remorse in committing it; and
revolting language used by persons whose natural purity
of taste and feeling are shown in the horror they feel and
express of the sort of compulsion under which they
are labouring.*

Admitting the truth of this description, as attested by
experience, the fact may be explained in some cases, as
we have seen, by the presence to the mind of real and
unreal objects of sense, each successively the subject of
belief, — this phenomenon itself possibly depending on the
doubleness of the brain and of the parts ministering to
perception, though we cannot obtain any certain proof
that such is the case.   But this explanation will not adequately apply to the instances where complete trains of
thought are perverted and deranged, while others are preserved in sufficiently natural course to become a sort of
watch upon the former.   Here we have no conjecture to
hazard other than that of supposing the two states of
mind to be never strictly coincident in time; — a view in

* It is impossible for one who has heard, ever to forget the strong
expressions of this kind occasionally used by patients themselves.   I
have seen a case of which the most marked feature was a frequent
and sudden outbreak of passion upon subjects, partly real, partly
delusive, but generally without obvious or sufficient reason at the
moment; — these excesses attended with loud screaming, execrations,
and acts of violence in striking or breaking things within reach.
Here the patient himself described to me the sort of separate
consciousness he had when these violent moods were upon him—his
desire, but feelings of inability to resist them—his satisfaction when
he felt them to be passing away.   It was a painfully exaggerated
picture of the struggle between good and ill.   " Contra miglior voler,
voler mal pugna."—*Dante.*

some sort sanctioned by what observation tells us of the inconceivable rapidity with which the mind actually shifts its state from one train of thought or feeling to another. In a former chapter I have treated at large on this subject, and shown our inability to measure by time these momentary passages of mental existence; crowding upon each other, and withal so interwoven into one chain, that consciousness, while it makes us aware of unceasing change, tells of no breach of continuity.

If the latter explanation be admitted, then the cases just mentioned come under the description of what has been termed *double consciousness;* where the mind passes by alternation from one state to another, each having the perception of external impressions and appropriate trains of thought, but not linked together by the ordinary gradations, or by mutual memory. I have seen one or two singular examples of this kind, but none so extraordinary as have been recorded by other authors.*   Their relations to the phenomena of sleep, of somnambulism, reverie, and insanity, abound in conclusions, of the deepest interest to every part of the mental history of man.

Even admitting, however, that these curiously contrasted states of mind are never strictly simultaneous, it is still a question whence their close concurrence is derived.   And, in the absence of any certainty on this very obscure subject, we may reasonably, perhaps, look to that part of our constitution in which manifest provision is made for unity of result from parts double in structure and function.

---

* One of the most remarkable cases of this nature is that narrated in Mr. Mayo's Physiology, 4th edition, p. 195.

This provision we know in many cases to be disturbed by accident, disease, or other less obvious cause; and though we cannot so well show this in regard to the higher faculties of mind, as in the instance of the senses and voluntary power, yet it is conceivable that there are cases where the two sides of the brain minister differently to these functions, so as to produce incongruity, where there should be identity or individuality of result.*

It is not easy to carry the argument beyond this form of simple question, without relinquishing that strict rule of inquiry which alone can be rightly pursued. But there are other points connected with this topic, of much interest to the physiology of man, and giving greater scope to research. For example, we have cause to suppose that

---

* It may be fitting to mention here a work of the late Dr. Wigan, published in 1844, entitled the "Duality of the Mind," and dedicated to me, in reference to the subject of this chapter. In this volume, the ingenious author has adopted, as the foundation of his reasoning, the various facts here stated; and has added numerous instances to the same effect. But he is much bolder in his inference from them; and plunges at once, as the title of his work implies, into the theory of a real *doubleness* or duality of mind; expressing it as a discovery which I might have reached had I ventured a little further in the same track. While admitting the frequent truth of what is so finely expressed by Lucretius, —

"Ardua dum metuunt amittunt vera viai,"

it is needful to add, that I can see no foundation for such doctrine. I believe that the suggestions offered above, though falling far short of an explanation of this obscure subject, yet come nearer to it than the opinion just alluded to. Surrounded as we are by mysteries, many of them insuperable by human reason, it is right to seek for, and record, whatever we can authenticate as facts; but unwise and injurious to push speculation beyond the closest induction from such observations.

there is in infancy a progressive education of the organs of sense, correcting the original perceptions they afford, defining the relations of the several senses, and giving unity of effect to impressions made on double organs.   Instances in proof of this are familiar to observation.   In like manner the education of the voluntary powers may be said not merely to extend the influence of the will to new muscular movements, but also to concentrate and individualise the powers of the mind in acts of volition, separating them more entirely from the involuntary actions of the same parts.   And carrying the argument further, we may suppose that the faculties of memory and combination are subject to the like education, tending always to give more proper and perfect unity to these functions than belongs to them in the outset of life, and thereby to establish more completely the conscious individuality of the being.

This view, if just in itself, is fertile in curious inferences, and serves better than any other to conciliate the phenomena of infancy with those of advancing age;—the progress from obscure or occasionally double perceptions, —from automatic or ill-regulated motions,—from imperfect and confused associations and impotence of recollection,—to that singleness in all acts of perception, volition, and memory which the mind attains in its healthy state, and which marks the intellectual character of man.   Here, however, we reach the many points at which human reason is forced to pause, before entering on paths too obscure for its further progress.

In the foregoing remarks I have spoken generally of

the brain as a double organ; referring only slightly to the
particular parts of this complicated structure; or to the
effects of morbid changes upon these severally, in altering the relation of the two sides, and the functions which
are perfect only from their entire correspondence.   The
excuse for this want of detail must be found in the very
incomplete knowledge we yet possess on the subject.
Notwithstanding all that has been obtained from comparative anatomy, pathology, and actual experiment (and large
has been of late years the gain from all these sources),
there are still few parts of the great nervous centres composing the brain, in which we can affirm with entire certainty the connexion between particular functions and
portions of structure.   On this subject I do not here
enlarge, as I shall have to speak more fully upon it in the
last chapter of this volume.   But the ignorance we are
still under, as to these particular relations, does not
materially affect the question before us.   The brain at
large is doubtless that part of the bodily organisation
which has closest connexion with all the higher functions
of our nature, and this is the essential point to be regarded,
as bearing upon the argument throughout.

In treating thus generally of the brain under its condition as a double organ, there has been no occasion to refer
to the doctrines of phrenology.   This system, indeed, in
recognising separate organs, perfectly alike and equivalent
to each other in each hemisphere, is bound more especially
to suppose that any casual disparity between the corresponding organs of the two sides must have effect in dis-
ordering the faculties therewith connected.   But the
course of argument just pursued is independent of these

particular assumptions. And, while seeking to enlarge
the foundation upon which we may rest further inquiry
into these organs, it does not profess more than to trace
one great condition of the cerebral structure — viz., that
of exact doubleness of parts — into some of its possible or
probable effects on the sensorial functions and the general
economy of life.

CHAP. IX.

ON PHRENOLOGY.

THE evidence as to the System of Phrenology of Gall, Spurzheim, and their followers, may be stated briefly as follows : —

The phrenologists rightly regard it as probable, or even as proved, that there is a certain plurality of parts in the total structure of the brain, corresponding to, and having connexion with, the different intellectual and moral faculties. The undoubted natural diversity of these faculties makes this probable, seeing that we must regard a certain organisation as ministering in the present life even to the higher powers of our nature. The partial and varying effects of accident, disease, or other less obvious change in the brain, in producing derangement of the mental functions, furnish more direct evidence, and such as we cannot refuse to admit. These effects are amongst the most remarkable which medical science affords in aid of our knowledge of man; and, whether with or without reference to phrenology, a careful record ought to be kept of all which are authenticated by trustworthy observers. They are materials of the highest value for future comparison and inference.

The phrenologists rightly represent the old classifications of mental phenomena (which are chiefly general expressions of function or capacity) as insufficient to

denote the various propensities and specialties of thought,
feeling, and action observed in different individuals, manifestly original to a certain extent, and forming, in conjunction with certain acquired or modified habits, the
particular character of each.

Thus far this doctrine has foundation in reason, but
not equally so its other parts. The multiform division
of these instinctive propensities (as under this view they
may fitly be called), though doubtless right in some
points, is arbitrary, inconsistent, or improbable in others;
and even in several material respects very differently
stated by phrenologists themselves. It was needful to
this method of inquiry, that some distribution of the
mental faculties and propensities should be taken as a
basis; but in the arrangement actually adopted there is a
strong flavour of human fiction, little in accordance with
the natural relations we are accustomed to admit. Viewed
as a whole, it is a sort of especial contradiction to the
" principe de la moindre action," so generally prevailing
throughout all parts of creation; and is yet further liable
o this peculiar objection, that the limitation of the list of
organs is hardly more reasonable than its extent. The
principle of division, if principle it can be called, might
have been carried greatly further. It scarcely admits of
boundary or exclusion.

Equally objectionable on other grounds is the remaining
part of the system; viz. the attribution of these mental
qualities or instincts to certain definite portions of the
brain, discoverable from without; and discoverable on the
presumption of the gross condition of quantity represent-
ing the intensity of quality, and the consequent vigour,

or even compulsory nature, of the actions thereon depending. This relation of mere bulk of substance to the perfection or intensity of a mental faculty (for it cannot otherwise be stated) is, *primâ facie*, very improbable; nor is it attested by observation of the structure of the brain, either viewed in mass, or by the more minute dissection and unfolding of parts, to which the authors of the system have themselves conducted us.

Admitting the great advance which has been made in the minute anatomy of the brain by these new modes of research, and appreciating the great merit of the observers, it is still difficult to see how the facts ascertained give support to their system of phrenology. The discovery of continuous and connecting fibres in the cerebral substance demonstrates, what must ever have been presumed, very complex relations of structure and function among the several parts of the brain. But neither in the nature nor distribution of these nervous fibres are there differences corresponding with the locality or limits of the organs which the doctrine describes; and the periphery of the brain, in particular, may be said to be singularly devoid of any indications of such division.* Nor, upon the actual

---

* It is true that the circumvolutions are the parts of the organ which offer the greatest variation, but these are in no respect more consistent with the scheme proposed to us. Nor have the more recent discoveries in this part of anatomy furnished, as far as I know, any sort of evidence to this effect. The writings of Tiedemann, Meckel, Wenzel, Retzius, &c., may be consulted on this subject, as well as some excellent English works of recent date. Among the later anatomical evidence applying to the question, I would mention the researches of M. Baillarger (1845), who, by a new method of unfolding and measuring the surfaces of the brain, has obtained results

principles of the system, is it easy to understand how the equally convoluted surface of the base of the hemispheres is to be disposed of, or the surfaces of the two hemispheres opposed to each other. The table of mental qualities is already over-crowded; yet here are portions of structure having a certain equality of claim to be admitted, though more remote from actual inspection.

The fact of the general smallness and deficient development of the cerebrum in congenital idiotcy—the ascertainment of the remarkable weight of the brain in certain persons of eminent intellect—and the great variety in the form of the cranium in different races of men—must be allowed as their best points in the argument; but, duly examined, these will be found insufficient in proof.* It seems, indeed, that many phrenologists admit different intensity of action in the several organs, as modifying the influence of size; and there can be no just reason for

which in his opinion prove that there is no relation whatever between the intelligence of animals and the extent of the cerebral surface; whether estimated absolutely, or in reference to the volume of the particular brain examined.

The function assigned by phrenologists to the great organ of the cerebellum is so important and distinct, that it ought to afford evidence of very decisive kind. But the contrary is true. Not merely is the proof on this point very uncertain; but there is much reason, as we shall notice elsewhere, to attribute other functions to it.

* In relation to the last of these three points, we find reason for affirming, upon the larger and more exact investigation of the crania of different races of men, that no general relation exists between their several forms and the mental qualities or endowments attached to them. The estimate of the latter point must ever be vague and uncertain; but the results obtained by different observers, and particularly by Professor Retzius, fully justify this remark.

refusing to them this qualification. Still the condition of size is the essential circumstance in the theory, and that which they are compelled to vindicate. It is this upon which the external demonstrations entirely depend, and without which the whole principle of action presumed must be viewed in a totally different light.*

But the phrenologists put this part of their doctrine upon the evidence of fact, and the fairness, or even conclusiveness, of this appeal cannot be denied. If the facts tallied uniformly with their assumptions — or even in a certain large proportion of cases, so as to make reasonable allowance for error or ambiguous result — the improbability must be laid aside of the mind being thus mechanically read from without, and the whole admitted as a new and wonderful truth.

Here then, by common admission, is a direct question of evidence, the amount and strictness of which are solely to be considered. And here, I think, it will be found that the phrenologists are yet wanting in what is needful to establish their system; notwithstanding all the observation and ingenuity which have been bestowed on its proof, and many singular coincidences between the theory and fact.

---

* The particular propensities of feeling and action expressed in the divisions and organs of the phrenologists, must, in every intelligible sense of the term, be deemed instincts, however modified or controlled by other instincts or actions opposed to them. And, accordingly, it has been sought to bring proof for the system from the relation to corresponding organs and habits in other animals. But, if not an objection, it is at least a singular anomaly under this view that certain insects, whose instincts are peculiarly complex, definite, and remarkable, as far as we can interpret them by our reason, should possess no cerebral organisation but that of nervous ganglia, so little concentrated as barely to warrant the name of brain.

Look at what they have in aid of their determinations, when the question concerns the relation between a certain outward form of the skull, and some faculty or quality of mind, alleged to be in correspondence with it. First, the equal chance of affirmative or negative as to each parti-- cular quality predicated. Secondly, the plea of a balance of some indications by others and opposing ones. Thirdly, the want of exact definition of many of these qualities or faculties; making it difficult to arrest for error, where there are so many ways of retreat. And fourthly, the incidental discovery of character by other and more ordi- nary methods of observation. I well know that the candid disciples of the system will not consciously avail them- selves of all these methods. Nevertheless each one of them has more or less been made use of; and, looking to the chances and facilities thus obtained, it may perhaps be affirmed that the number of true predictions in phreno- logy is less miraculous than it would be, were this number not to occur. Here we have a question purely of fact, and the statement just made may be disputed as such. But I think it will be found by those who look fairly into the matter, that the coincidences are not more frequent or remarkable than the assured average of chances would make them to be; and that the contradictions are more numerous than would be likely to happen were the system one of established truth.

In these few remarks I have chiefly sought to put the several points of the question into a clear light. It is obvious that these points are widely different in them- selves, and differ much in their degree of probability.

Respecting the evidence of that which is cardinal to the
system, viz. the power of discovery of strong faculties and
instincts of action by the external configuration of the
skull, the fairest test would be found, not in vague and
ill-defined moral propensities, respecting the site of many
of which phrenologists are far from being agreed among
themselves; but in a few simple and well-marked faculties, such as those of numerical calculation, languages, or
music; which have none others in obvious opposition to
them, and the degree of perfection in which can be clearly
defined by observation. It is true that the phrenologists
appeal to these particular cases in their evidence, and
many examples doubtless occur where such appeal has
been made good. But the doctrine requires that it should
more uniformly be so than those will admit, who fairly
look at any large number of instances in which this system
has been put to proof under their own inspection.*

In the present state of our knowledge of the brain, and
of its relation to the mental functions, an impartial view
of phrenology requires, not that the principle should be
dismissed from view, but that great abatement should be
made of its pretensions as a system. To say the least, it
is chargeable with what Lord Bacon has called " an over-
early and peremptory reduction into acts and methods,"

---

* During some intercourse with Gall, and more frequently with
Spurzheim (both remarkable men, and deeply impressed with the
truth of their opinions), I had several occasions of noticing the failure
of their judgment upon the particular faculties mentioned above; as
well as in other cases where the peculiarity of external conformation,
or of some given quality of mind, made it almost needful that the
doctrine should rightly indicate the relations upon which it professes to be based.

and with the adoption of various conclusions, not warranted by any sufficient evidence. But on a subject thus obscure in all its parts, and where our actual knowledge is still limited to detached facts or presumptions, there is enough to justify the opinion being kept before us, as one of the outlines to which future observations may legitimately apply ; — not fettered, as they now are, by the trammels of a premature arrangement.*

---

* I think it right to refer here to an article in No. XVII. of the British and Foreign Medical Review, in which, with relation to this Chapter, as well as to other and larger treatises on the subject, the argument for phrenology is very ably and fairly stated.

CHAP. X.

ON INSTINCTS AND HABITS.

IT would be difficult to add any thing new to what has been written on the great question of Instincts, and yet the main points continue unresolved. Witnesses at every moment of the phenomena of animal life which belong to this class — phenomena certain as facts, numberless in variety, and more curious as the observation of them is more minute — our knowledge on the subject must still be regarded as elementary. Men of thought in every age have felt their wonder, and been solicitous to penetrate along an avenue, which seems to lead to the higher myste-ries of creative and sustaining power. But the path, obscure even at its entrance, is speedily closed to us. Modern science, with all its aids to research, has effected little more than the better description and distinction of facts ; and in obtaining this result has brought fresh pro-blems and difficulties into view, showing yet more to be done, in proportion as the scope and methods of the in-quiry are better defined.*

---

* Bayle has justly termed the actions of beasts, "Un des plus pro-fonds abîmes, sur quoi notre raison peut s'exercer." And, in truth, the relation of these actions to the higher reason and more limited instincts of man, while illustrating some points, does in others make still wider this great chasm in human knowledge.

Definition, of course, has been busy with the subject,
and under a wide range of description. We have an example of this in the singular difference of analogy by
which Laplace and Cuvier have severally defined animal
instincts. The " Affinité animale analogue à celle qui
rapproche les molécules des cristaux," is an expression of
the former, far less happy than the " Somnambulisme " of
Cuvier—the determination of instinctive actions by innate
perceptions or images ever present in succession on the
sensorium. But it will be obvious, on slight consideration,
how far these and all other analogies fall short of any
true theory of Instincts. Nor can we carry the expression
of our knowledge beyond certain series of facts, which it
is impossible to contravene, and certain relations definite
enough to furnish a ground for further inquiry.

The main point, to which all others are subordinate, is
the essential difference between instinctive actions and
those of reason. Though ingenious men have sought to
undermine this distinction,—some by raising instinct to
the character of reason, others by submitting the latter to
a metaphysical necessity, intelligible only as an instinct,—
yet are the examples so decisive of separate source and
manner of operation in these two classes of actions, that
no subtlety of argument is of avail against them. The
absolute hereditary nature of instincts,—their instant or
speedy perfection, prior to all experience or memory,
—their provision for the future, without prescience of
it,—the preciseness of their objects, extent, and limitation,—and the distinctness and permanence of their
character for each species,—these are the more general
facts on which our definition must be founded. The

examples illustrating it are endless, and connected with every form and grade of animal life, — from the few and subordinate instincts of man, to those wonderful groups and series of automatic actions which constitute the total existence of the lower orders of creation. The conclusion to which these examples concur becomes irresistible. We can adopt no definition of instinct and reason which does not indicate their separate nature.

This distinction adopted, we might seem to have obtained a fair basis for further research. Yet, going a step beyond, we find ourselves involved in the arduous questions already mentioned, — scarcely one of them yet wholly solved, some of them in their nature incapable of solution. Even the line of separation between instinct and reason, which seems so clearly designated in nature, becomes vague and indistinct when we seek to carry it through all the functions of animal life. I cannot do more here than indicate the main questions open on this debateable ground. To discuss them fully, and with the illustrations so largely furnished by the natural history of instincts, would require not a chapter but a volume.

Having, as far as needful, denoted the distinctive character of instincts, the first question concerns their relative distribution throughout the different parts of organic existence. At the one extremity of this great scale we have the blending of intelligence and instinct, as we find it in the human being and the higher animals, — at the other, the connexion of animal instincts with those of vegetable life. Excluding the latter topic, however curious, from the discussion, the immediate inquiry regards the gradation of instincts through the long series

of animal life. At whichsoever end of the scale we begin,
—whether we consider instincts simply supplementary to
intelligence, or, (as is more congruous with the order of
natural succession,) reason to be superinduced upon instincts,—equally do we find these two great faculties
manifested in an inverse ratio to each other, throughout
every part of the animal creation in which both exist. In
man instincts, properly so called, form the *minimum* in
relation to reason. They are few in number, and difficult
of definition from their connexion with his higher mental
functions. They multiply continually, and become more
distinct in character, as we descend in the scale; their
completeness, in reference to the life of the individual,
increasing in the same ratio as the intelligence becomes
less. A point doubtless exists in the series, though perhaps indeterminable, where they wholly govern all the
acts of life; becoming identical with existence itself, and
closely allied to corresponding functions of the vegetable
world. Any semblance of exception to the general law
depends, probably, on our imperfect knowledge of its
operation in particular cases.

In this proportion, then, and manner of distribution
through the various grades of animal life, we find the distinctive character of these automatic actions marked
almost as clearly as by the nature of the acts themselves.
And, by the confirmation thus obtained of the natural
separation and contrast of instinct and reason, we are
carried at once to the question of the origin of the former,
even before discussing those intimate relations by which
they are so singularly, yet beneficially, blended in the
economy of life. Both faculties of action are derived from

a higher power than the beings possessing them, and in this one sense may be deemed the same. But one faculty is given to be consciously and voluntarily used, with large capacity for improvement, and with other endowments which fit it for the most exalted purposes ;—the other is uniform, determinate, and having origin and guidance wholly apart from the will. Whence comes this origin and guidance ? *

The question has naturally engaged the attention of philosophers of every age ; and we find annexed to it the great names of Bacon, Newton, Descartes, and Locke, in succession to those of higher antiquity. They have been followed again by many eminent writers of modern times ; and metaphysics and physiology have been brought into close alliance in seeking for a solution. The main point in the argument is that distinctly propounded by Sir Isaac Newton in his 31st Query ;—Can we otherwise explain animal instincts than by supposing that the Deity himself is virtually the active and present moving principle in them? This opinion Newton adopts; seeking to separate the doctrine, and the ubiquity of the Deity implied in it,

---

* I purposely refrain here from any allusion to the much-argued questions of Liberty and Necessity. It would ill assort with a subject, already so difficult in itself, to involve it in this ancient labyrinth of verbal disputes. The questions of most moment may be discussed independently of any such bearing.

If we might go to poetry for illustration of such topics, there are some lines in Pope's "Essay on Man," which describe, with a vigour not unlike that of Dryden, the peculiar character of Instinct : —

> " But honest Instinct comes a volunteer,
> Sure never to o'ershoot, but just to hit,
> While still too wide, or short, is human wit."

from that grosser Pantheism into which so many philosophers of every age have fallen while dealing with these
subtle questions.*

Unless, indeed, we merge both reason and instinct in
this common chaos, it is difficult to avoid the general conception just stated. The instinctive action has an express
object of which the animal has no prior cognisance — to
attain which its living organisation goes through certain
changes and movements, definite, identical, and constant
for each one of the species. Where reason exists, even in
the animals nearest to man, it is placed in subordination to
this more absolute power; blending with and modifying,
but never annulling its influence. Here, then, all proper
volition, or act of the individual, is excluded; and the
Creator of the organisation becomes, in every sense intelligible to us, the motive power. We may choose to say,
that the organisation itself is so; but to such phrase, duly
examined, we can attach no real meaning, nor can we
substantiate it by any manner of proof. At this point, in
fact, the argument, as concerns human reason, is at an end.
We cannot conceive the intervention of other agency; but
neither are we able to reach the comprehension of that
Supreme Power which thus unceasingly sustains the life
it has created. The creation and the maintenance by
instinctive action, are to us mysteries of the same nature;
and so far alike, indeed, to our comprehension, that the

* Lord Brougham, in his "Dialogues on Instinct," published years
ago, espouses the same opinion, and vindicates it with great ability on
the same grounds. I have not room here to allude to the various
opinions of the numerous writers who have discussed this and other
points connected with the theory of Instincts.

sole analogy we can conceive to the latter is in that power
on which organisation and life depend.*

The instincts of the Bee have been most frequently
selected for illustration on this subject; and not without
reason, as regards the singular economy of social life in
this animal, and those equally marvellous instincts of
structure by which, for thousands of years, their cells have
been fabricated according to laws of the most rigid mathematical exactness: In reality, this instance is not more
wonderful than a thousand others with which natural history makes us familiar. The objects, means, and results,
differ for every particular species; but by each they are
accomplished with the same admirable certitude and completeness. Be it the Ant, the Spider, the Salmon, the
Swallow, the Beaver, or the Dog, the argument and inference are strictly alike. They all equally enforce the
question just stated as to the proximate cause of the
actions thus attached to different animal organisms; while
at the same time they repress every rational hope of
attaining its solution. †

---

* There is one point of view under which we must regard organisation and instinct with reference to a common and single origin.
Wherever there is organisation, even under the simplest form, there
we are sure to find instinctive action, more or less in amount, destined
to give the appropriate effect to it. This is true throughout every
part of the animal series, from Man and the Quadrumana down to the
lowest form of infusorial life. When we consider how vast this scale
is — crowded with more than a hundred thousand recognised species,
exclusively of those which fossil geology has disclosed to us — we
may well be amazed by this profuse variety of instinctive action; as
multiplied in kind as are the organic forms with which it is associated,
and all derived from one common Power.

† It is worthy of note, in farther proof of the inverse perfection of

Quitting this question then, as beyond our reach, we come to others, difficult indeed, but more within the compass of our knowledge.— Are intelligence and instinct, thus differing in their relative proportion in man as compared with all other animals, yet the same in kind and manner of operation in both? To this question we must give an affirmative answer. The expression of Cuvier regarding the faculty of reason in lower animals— " Leur intelligence exécute des opérations du même genre,"— is true in its full sense. We can in no manner define reason so as to exclude acts which are at every moment present to our observation, and which we find in many instances to contravene the natural instincts of the species. On the other side we may justly affirm that the instincts of man, wherever we can truly distinguish them, are the same in principle and manner of operation as those of other animals — common to the species ; definite in their objects and the means adapted to their fulfilment; and separate from reason, though continually governed and limited by it. We shall hereafter see the difficulties of distinction and exact definition which embarrass this part of the question; but meanwhile it is enough to specify the resemblances just stated.

In considering this curious question of the relation of human instincts to those of lower animals, a valuable distinction may be derived from looking to their respective

intellect and instinct, that the class of insects in whom these instinctive functions are most strikingly manifested appears, as far as we can judge in such a matter, to rank very low in the scale of intelligence. All the social acts so wonderfully exhibited in different species of the Hymenoptera and Neuroptera are liable to this remark.

development in species and individuals.   In other animals
instincts are chiefly, or entirely, those of the species, uniform and permanent; with far less of intelligence in any
case to modify or control them, and this at a certain point
disappearing altogether.   In man they have more of individual character, are far less numerous and definite in
relation to the physical conditions of life, more various and
extensive in regard to his moral nature; yet still subject,
as such, to the control of his intellectual powers.   It
seems the proper destination of reason, as bestowed by his
Creator, to acquire mastery over the instinctive conditions
of his nature; to cultivate some, to subdue others, to give
due proportion and direction to all.

   The functions of organic life furnish a large class of
actions common to man with the inferior animals.   These
functions — mainly independent of the will, and uniform in
their character and course — may seem on first view closely
allied to the instincts which connect animals with the
external world, ministering to their food, habitation, pro-
tection, and the propagation of the species.   Yet is this
analogy not such as to justify our placing them under the
same class.   We find the nervous system of organic life
attached to parts of well-defined structure; fulfilling internal functions essential to existence itself; and by actions
which, except in certain cases, are scarcely ever the subject of consciousness.   Instincts, on the other hand, have
relation chiefly to things without — they are bound up
closely in every part with animal life and voluntary motions, through actions of the same organs — the actions
themselves continually graduate into each other; in some
cases by original association of function, in others by the

influence of habit giving to voluntary acts much of the character and force of instinctive propensities.

This argument may be carried a step further. We find in the simple functions of organic life — the vital processes of respiration, circulation, nutrition, secretion, &c. —a certain community in all classes of animals, as respects the objects and the manner of fulfilling them. The differences of the organisation, so applied, are often more of outward aspect than reality ; and, in many cases, similarity of structure in these parts is carried down with wonderful precision from the higher grades of animal life to those far lower in the scale.* Instincts, on the contrary, are infinitely diversified in their methods, even where the general purposes, as generation, nourishment, habitation, defence, &c. are essentially the same. This variety is equal and

---

* The law of Unity of Composition—(though, perhaps, carried too far by some physiologists, and to be considered only as a co-ordinate with that other great principle, which determines with equal precision the *diversity* in the forms of life)—has a substantial reality in nature. It is ever suggesting analogies and relations of structure, to which even identity of function failed in directing attention before ; and which exist in some cases where the function is wanting, to which the particular type of structure applies.

In the two treatises of Professor Owen,—on the "Archetype and Homologies of the Vertebrate Skeleton," and on the "Nature of Limbs,"—we have the most perfect illustration of the doctrine of Typical Forms in its connexion with that of special adaptation,—a connexion clearly established in nature, and which must ever be kept in view as one of the bases of inquiry on this subject. Few laws in physical science have acquired more certainty, or contributed more to just conclusions, than that which designates the progress from the *General* to the *Special* in every part of organised creation.

P

relative to the multiplied conditions of the objects upon
which they act.   Every species of organised being (for the
expression must be extended even to vegetable life) has
its peculiar relations to things without—definite, original,
and, as far as we know, perpetual to the species.   The
instincts, properly so called, of animal life, include a large
proportion of these relations.   Their peculiarity for each
species, and perpetuity through successive generations, are
among the wonderful characters inscribed by Providence,
and recognised but not deciphered by man.

The simple organism of life, then, even if denominated
instinct in a large sense of the word, is not really identical
with that agency more properly so called, which may be
said to take the place and part of reason in the animal.
Whatever ambiguity arises from the automatic character
of the acts in each case, neither the structure concerned in
these functions, nor the manner of their operation, furnishes
any proof of identity in the principle of power.   Nor,
again, can we admit the perfection of the senses in different animals, as coming properly under the definition of
instincts.   That exquisite sensibility of sight, touch, smell,
or hearing, which we find in numerous instances so far
transcending what is possessed by man, must be regarded
not as instinctive action itself, but as the instrumentality
by which such action is directed and fulfilled.*

---

* These points are ably discussed in an article of the " North
American Review " for July 1846, — a work to which I most willingly
allude, as having been remarkable throughout its whole career for
the great excellence of its philosophical articles, as well as those of
literary criticism.

We now come more directly to the question regarding these two faculties of Reason and Instinct, as they are developed and co-exist in man himself, without reference to other parts of the animal world. The inquiry is not less difficult from this limitation. The association of instincts with the higher intellect of man, does in truth render all its manifestations more equivocal and obscure. After all that we have said on the distinction between the two powers, it is not easy to affirm where the one ends and the other begins — to interpret rightly the numerous cases whose automatic and habitual actions, scarcely to be distinguished from instincts, blend themselves with those of reason and volition, and, in the union, accomplish some of the most important functions of life—to solve the doubts which arise from each class of actions being carried on by the same organic apparatus — or to define, with reference to the question, those congenital propensities, intellectual and moral, which so strongly mark individual character, and influence the whole course of human life.

All these questions, it will be seen, tend to run into metaphysical or verbal ambiguities, whence it is not easy to extricate them. Take, for instance, the last of the topics just named. How are we to distinguish these propensities of thought, feeling, and action from true instincts? Like them, they are innate — they modify, often control or compel, the whole course of life—in some cases they are felt as opposed to the reason of the individual, yet dominant over it — in extreme cases, they become a sort of madness by opposition to the reason of the species. If

instincts are to be defined as a necessity of animal existence, these propensities can hardly be excluded from the
class; though, in their connexion with the intellect and
will, differing so widely from the mere physical instincts
which we find lower down in the scale of life.

Or again, if in a general sense admitting them, how
are we to define, in reference to this subject, those various
forms of intuitive mental perception, the question as to
the recognition of which has caused so much discussion in
the modern schools of philosophy? The very diversity of
names used to express these conditions (" innate or fundamental ideas," "categories of the understanding," "intuitive conceptions," &c.) will show how difficult it is to
describe their nature, or to express their common relation
to the individuality of the mind.*

Some additional facility may be given to this inquiry
by adopting the division into physical and mental instincts;
as marking a very important distinction of character and
office. Still, however, we remain under the influence of
definitions ; nor would this distinction draw a line, as
might at first appear, between man and other animals.
Those nearest to man in the scale (and we have no means
of marking the point where the analogy ceases) exhibit
individualities of intelligence and feeling, in connexion
with the instincts of the species, which we can in no wise

* The writings of Reid, Kant, and other authors of later date, will
furnish many other phrases to the same effect — all labouring to give
some certain specification to facts in themselves equivocal and obscure.
The *Noumena* of Kant, in contradistinction to *Phenomena*, is, perhaps
from its generality, the happiest of the terms so employed.

distinguish from the innate human propensities just described—independent of reason, though in action so closely associated with it. In adopting, then, this distinction of mental and physical instincts, every question is still subordinate to the more general definition of instinctive action already given.

I have already alluded to the functions of organic life, common to man with other animals, and the circumstances which distinguish these from Instincts. But there is another class of actions, in which man is especially concerned, and which are of more doubtful interpretation. I allude to those automatic or involuntary movements of the body, consequent upon the presence of mental emotions or passions; of which the acts of laughing and crying furnish the most characteristic and frequent examples. Their familiarity will not disguise from the philosophic observer the remarkable part they bear in the physical as well as moral history of man. These outward expressions of inward emotion—common to the human species in all its races and varieties — are evidently designed in the constitution, and with express reference to the social state of man. Their equivalents in other animals are scanty and obscure. We may wonder at the manner in which they are testified; through the involuntary or convulsive action of parts which habitually subserve to voluntary motion; or by the increased secretion from a gland which has other specific uses in the economy of the eye. It may seem strange, too, that while they often directly contravene the will, these outward expressions are capable of being perfectly counterfeited by it. The actor simulates, and through

the very same muscles, the convulsive laughter or sobs
which are excited at other times by certain ideas or emotions of mind, despite every effort to restrain them.*

We may best obtain explanation to satisfy this wonder,
by considering that the objects to be fulfilled required
these expressions of feeling to be external, and readily
obvious to sense; and further, that they should be closely
associated with those organs and functions through which
the will exercises its control. Thus regarded, we find in
the method as well as object of these acts, one of those
wonderful provisions of our nature, by which functions,
seemingly dissimilar or opposed, are made to minister to
each other, and to a common end.

The whole subject of the physical expressions of mental
emotion — of the passion, feelings, and even intellectual
states — is, in truth, one of deep interest both to physiology and the philosophy of mind. The facts which have
been examined and classed under the name of Physiog-
nomy, come in close relation to it; and they all connect
themselves with the question before us, not only by the
instinctive character of the acts of expression, but also by
the sort of intuitive perception with which they are re-

---

* It is worthy of notice, that the external expressions appropriated
to certain feelings undergo change at different periods of life, and in
different constitutions. The child cries and sobs from fear or pain;
the adult more generally from sudden grief, or warm affection, or
sympathy with the feeling of others.

Poetry, the language of emotion, has in every age busied itself in
the delineation of these outward expressions of feeling, and the
greatest poets have seized on the finest shades. The Δακρυοεν γελασασα
will be remembered by every reader of Homer; exquisitely para-
phrased by our own great poet in his " Richard the Second."

ceived by others. It is impossible, in reasoning on this topic, to define exactly what is due to habit, imitation, or experience. But that there is some cause concerned, more instant and more universal than any of these, we can hardly refuse to believe, under whatever name we describe it. The difficulty of definition here, as in every case where man is the subject, arises from that closer blending of the intellect and will with every physical act — *concurrence* in some cases, *conflict* in others — which makes it almost impossible even for the consciousness to distinguish between what is instinctive, what voluntary, in this part of our nature.

Certain acts of early infancy have been generally cited under the class of human instincts, and, it may be, rightly. But it must be observed that if we refer the first sucking of the infant (probably a simple reflex action following an impression on the nerves of sense) to the same source as the instincts of the spider or bee, we virtually admit all the complex and wonderful acts of the latter as being simply the sequel to impressions on the sentient nerves — a view, as we have seen, which it would be difficult to maintain, though propounded by some physiologists as a partial solution of the question.

The class of Instincts belonging to the propagation of the species are, in every part of the animal kingdom, among the most remarkable of which we have any cognisance.*

* Our knowledge of all that relates to the reproduction of species in animals, though largely advanced of late by new facts, is still but of secondary kind, as respects the solution of this great problem of nature. The more minute examination of the successive changes in

Strongly defined in all other animals, they receive in man the same modification as do his other instinctive propensities; blending themselves closely and variously with the moral and intellectual parts of his nature; and in this union evolving many of those feelings and finer characters of human life, which best distinguish it from the brute part of creation. An instinct of absolute necessity in its object, is thus rendered a principle of our moral constitution, and connects itself with all our moral responsibilities; while at the same time it furnishes materials for those powers of imagination, taste, and perception of beauty, which, if not absolutely peculiar to man, are at least his possession in degree infinitely above all that can be admitted into the comparison.*

the ovum and germinal vesicle, — the discoveries regarding the structure and development by cells, — those equally remarkable just made by Mr. Newport as to the peculiar actions of the Spermatozoa, — the singular facts recently determined respecting fissiparous and gemmiparous propagation, — and the researches as to the special phenomena which have been classed under the names of Metagenesis and Parthenogenesis, — all these and other discoveries bring us only to the threshold of the question regarding a power which can thus (sometimes under sexual conditions, sometimes independently of them,) evolve and reproduce through individuals an interminable series of those organised forms, instincts, and other attributes which belong to the particular species. Closely examined, it may be that this is not a greater mystery than the functions of nutrition, reparation, &c.; for beyond a certain point we can attach no understanding to any of these actions. But in studying the laws of generation, we seem, whatever the reality, to be making a nearer approach to the sources of that creative power, which is ever reproducing the same forms through laws of organisation intelligible to us only in their effects.

* Of all writers whom I know, Dr. Macculloch is the one who argues with most force on behalf of the faculties and feelings of other animals as compared with man. In his posthumous volumes on

Amidst the various difficulties belonging to the proper definition of instincts, we have yet to see what aid can be furnished to us by anatomy;—whether there is any speciality of structure so far associated with them as to designate what acts are of this kind, what of another? And we naturally look to Comparative Anatomy, that fertile source of knowledge, for furtherance in the research. The evidence, both positive and negative, which it affords in questions of this nature, is often such as can be drawn from no other source.

It is obvious that this inquiry wholly concentrates itself on the nervous system, as the sole part of the animal economy which can be supposed to give origin or excitement to actions of this description. Though absolutely unable to show, or even to conceive, how nervous matter should minister to these particular functions, or to others which it is better proved to maintain; yet if we found certain portions of it invariably connected with certain well-marked instincts, and never present where they are not, we might fairly affirm that we had gained some ground in advance.

But this amount of knowledge is far from being yet attained. We have already seen that we cannot consider as true instincts those automatic functions which form part of the great system of organic life; and here, therefore, we must not look for that portion of nervous structure which serves to proper instinctive action. The

Natural Theology—a work of great ability and learning, but defaced by much perverted taste,—will be found several chapters devoted especially to this subject.

question, however, becomes more difficult when we apply
it to the cerebro-spinal system, and the nerves ministering
to sensation and voluntary motion, as well as to the reflex
automatic actions which form so important a part of the
economy of life.   Instincts are undoubtedly carried into
effect through these organs and acts; and up to this
point, therefore, the inquiry is answered.   But it is still a
knowledge of the instruments only we have obtained; and
even limiting ourselves to the anatomical question, we
are led to look further for some nervous centres, appropriate to these extraordinary faculties, and giving power
at least, if not direction, to their several manifestations.
That there is some such association in the case of Instincts, as well as of the intellectual faculties, we are
bound by analogy to suppose probable, even though we
cannot denote the situation of any especial nervous organs
destined to this function.

The most distinct knowledge we here possess is indeed
of a negative kind.   It is certain that neither the cerebral
lobes nor cerebellum are necessary, or directly concerned
in instinctive actions, inasmuch as these peculiar organs
are confined to the Vertebrata, and wholly wanting to
large classes of animals whose instincts are highly developed.   Excluding them, the closest analogy we can
obtain in seeking for nervous centres of these functions, is
probably that of the ganglia appertaining to the organs
of special sensation.   Comparative anatomy, indeed, concurs with analogy in leading us to conjecture that the
ganglionic structure (using the term in its common application) is the nervous apparatus most directly instrumental
to instincts.   The examination of the nervous system, as

we find it in descending the scale of animal life, strengthens this inference, by showing the great development of these parts, their definite arrangement in each species, their prodigious variety in different classes of the animal kingdom. It is true that we reach a point, proximate to the vegetable world, where actions that we must call instinctive are still found in organised beings, unpossessed, as far as we can see, of any nervous tissue. Even here, however, we have no proof that nervous matter does not exist, in some form equivalent to the necessities of this low grade of being. The most subtle use of the microscope is unavailing when we reach these elementary points (the αμερη ελαχιστα) of organised structure.

Admitting this general conclusion, which needs no illustration to those familiar with Comparative Anatomy, we still have advanced but little in the inquiry. Even in the limited number of cases where we can associate some particular instinct with a specialty of nervous structure, we are utterly unprovided with reason or conjecture as to the manner of relation. It is a bare fact, unfruitful of present inferences. If we could prove with assurance that certain nervous ganglia were indispensable to the instincts of the bee, what clue should we thereby gain to the construction of the hexagonal cell, or to the perfect mathematical figure of the rhomb which closes it, or what insight into the complex social instincts of this wonderful insect? The connexion here of the material organs with the animal action is as obscure as that of the cerebral organisation with the intellectual faculties of man, and equally insuperable by research.

Nor do we gain more certain knowledge by looking to

the reflex functions of the nervous system, as giving cause
and direction to instinctive actions, singularly important
though these functions are. It is true that in various
classes of animals, as the insects, whose instincts are
strongly marked, we have the proofs of reflex nervous
influence in many striking phenomena of life. We have
proof also that many remarkable instincts depend for their
exercise on the perfection of the senses ministering to
them, of which the exquisite sensibility of the organs of
touch and smell in numerous animals affords illustration.
It is further true, that various actions of voluntary organs
become thoroughly habitual by long repetition, and approach to the instinctive character as far as the will is
concerned. Observations have been adduced to show that
some instincts are impaired by injuries to the brain and
spinal marrow; and the less ambiguous experiments of
Huber and Latreille are well known, in which, by
depriving bees and ants of their antennæ, they destroyed,
or rendered inert, certain of the most peculiar instinctive
powers of these insects.

These several facts, however, while they show the necessity of the organs of sense and nerves of reflex action, as
instruments of the faculty, lead to no certain inference
beyond. They do not explain to us how the uniformity
and precision of specific instincts, throughout the vast
variety of animal life, can be maintained by impressions on
the senses from external objects and agents, themselves in
a state of unceasing change. That instincts are often
modified, sometimes controlled, by external causes pressing
upon them, must at once be admitted. But this fact

comes before us rather as the exception, than the course or rule of action. Or again, if we are referred to internal organisation, as in part the source of these impressions (and the instincts of generation may seem to justify this reference), we have still to ask where this organisation is, and in what it consists? The evidence, in truth, on every part of this subject, is rather that of partial analogy than positive knowledge. And when we seem to have gained some step in advance, it is but a point from which to see more clearly the difficulties beyond. We may have crossed the bar of the river, but there lies before us the unfathomable gulf into which it flows. *

It may reasonably surprise any one new to the subject, that so large a part of the foregoing discussion should be occupied by the statement of difficulties, while so little is effected for their solution. The fact, which must be fully admitted, belongs to the very nature of the inquiry; and it may be added also, to the principle I have pursued throughout this volume, of distinguishing, as fairly as I

---

* Some further knowledge, though still limited in its scope, may perhaps be gained from observation of the relative development of nerves, connected with the particular functions by which specific instincts are maintained, as in the case of the electrical fishes. And such comparison may be aided in many cases by notice of those remarkable changes which the nerves of certain animals undergo in their natural transformations of state, as in the change from the *Larva* to the *Pupa* state, and again to that of the *Imago*, in insects. Here, however, our inference must be limited by the actual diversity of life in these different states; implying changes of function for each, apart from any relation to those trains of action in which we understand instincts to consist.

can, between what is our certain knowledge in each case, and what is doubtful, speculative, or unattainable. The subject of Instincts, as separate from the mere history of phenomena, includes so much that can only come under the latter description, that we may find in this circumstance a sufficient reason for the manner in which its discussion has been conducted.

We must at once admit, that by connecting the subject of Habits with it, we do not lessen the difficulties referred to. Yet there are so many points of relation between the two topics, whether by resemblance or contrast, that I have been led to place them in the same chapter for their mutual illustration; and with the further view of indicating, by some general remarks on Habit, the great importance of the subject, both to physiology and the treatment of disease.

Any definition of Habit, general enough to include all the applications of the term, would be of little practical value; for even vegetable life might come within its scope.* Limiting the view, however, to animal life, and for obvious reasons, chiefly to that of Man, we find its distinctive character to consist mainly in this, — that acts,

---

* The existence of a principle of Habit in vegetable life must be conceded, if we adopt as its definition a change in the character of natural functions, without obvious alteration of structure, in effect of the repetition of certain external actions upon them. Among other experiments affirmative on this point may be noticed those of De Candolle; in which, by artificial methods of altering the times of light and darkness, he succeeded in some plants in producing a correspondent change of the time of opening and closing their flowers. It is worthy of note, that the *Sensitive Plant* underwent the greatest change in the shortest period of time.

whether of body or mind, whether single or in series, do, if often repeated, tend to recur afterwards in the same order of time and succession; — this tendency being proportionate to the frequency and uniformity of repetition; modified by the will, but sometimes contravening and overcoming it. Habits are obviously designed to fulfil purposes essential to animal life. They link together into particular series acts which originally are single and insulated; giving them through this combination a power and efficiency which else were wholly wanting. As is the case with every other faculty of our nature, that which, in the majority of cases, serves to expedient or necessary uses, becomes exceptionally a source of injury or disorder. The effect of habit in giving an automatic character, almost like an instinct, to certain groups of muscular actions — as in speaking, walking, and the other numerous and complex movements of the limbs—is absolutely necessary to human existence, and admirably suited to this necessity. But other habits may be created in the very same organs, by accident or hurtful use, which entirely frustrate these purposes, and become causes of disorder in the animal economy. This distinction still more strikingly applies to mental habits. Some minister directly to the power and integrity of the intellect, or to the moral discipline of the mind. Others are faulty and injurious associations, which by repetition become almost compulsory in their nature, and usurp the place and prerogative of reason.

In fixing the relation between Habits and Instincts, an essential point is their respective relation to the will. Instincts are independent of it in their origin; though afterwards, in many cases, modified by its influence. Habit

in the sense in which we have used the term, expresses the
tendency towards automatic character in acts, which were
originally governed, more or less, by voluntary power.
It is well worthy of note how closely the results continually
approach to each other, though thus remote or even opposite in their source.   This resemblance—one of the many
examples of the great law of continuity — while it imparts
much interest to all that regards the relation of these
functions, adds materially to the difficulty of distinguishing
them in particular cases.   We need to recur often to the
definition of Instincts—to their instant perfection, their
sameness and permanence for the species, the preciseness
of their objects, extent, and limitation — to separate them
duly from those effects of habit, which are ever present to
observation.   The actions belonging to the latter—various
and vague in their origin, differing in individuals of the
species, ever liable to be altered or cancelled by the incidents of life, and more or less under the control of intelligence and will — these actions obviously form a separate
part of the scheme of animal existence; and in Man especially, seem designed to represent the attributes of instinct, in the increased facility and certainty they give to
the results of reason and voluntary power.

The closest approximation of Habits and Instinct is
undoubtedly shown in the tendency of the former to
become hereditary — a fact variously proved both as to
bodily and mental habits; and equally curious and important in reference to the whole economy of animal life.
The influence of this principle in the case of domesticated
animals is too well known to need examples in illustration.
Man is here the powerful agent in superimposing habits

upon instincts — modifying and contrasting the latter for his especial purposes, though never annihilating them.* He is himself subject to the same natural laws, operating on every part of his intellectual and social state. The tendency to become hereditary exists not solely in the habits of health, but even in various effects of disorder and disease; though under conditions which from their multiplicity and complex relations it is not easy to define. In a chapter " On Hereditary Disease," in my former work, I have stated numerous examples to this effect; and could greatly add to them, were this necessary. It is rendered certain indeed, by instances derived from every part of organic life, that congenital peculiarities, or deviations from the natural type, may become hereditary as varieties of the species. And we have evidence equally certain that peculiarities derived from the conditions of life, if common to many individuals, may also be propagated and become hereditary in a community or race.

The topic before us, in its relations to the animal creation at large, blends itself with certain of the most profound problems of natural science; those, namely, which relate to the generic and specific distinctions of

---

* There is still great room for research on this interesting subject. The opposite questions equally merit examination. — In what time, through what means, and under what limitation, may habits be rendered hereditary? — and, to what extent, and in what period and manner, are the instincts of the species resumed, upon withdrawal of the conditions creating these habits? It will be readily seen that such inquiries, pursued towards exact results, require great minuteness of observation, and long periods of time, for their solution. But the zeal and accuracy now carried into every branch of Natural History are the best augury of eventual success.

animal life; and the extent to which natural changes, propagated and extended through successive generations, may have effect in producing these distinctive characters. Every naturalist is familiar with the questions that have arisen on this subject, and with the theory of change and transmutation which some have sought to raise on this general foundation — setting at nought, in so doing, the old doctrine and definition of species; and labouring to prove that, if unlimited time be conceded, these distinctions may all merge in more general laws of internal change and progression. Under this principle it is assumed that acquired habits, becoming hereditary, assume the character of specific instincts; and are associated with changes of form, simultaneously proceeding from the same causes; the whole forming a scheme of progressive transmutation throughout every part of created life.*

---

* The reference here will be obvious to the doctrine of which Lamarck has been a chief advocate among the continental naturalists, and which has lately gained some ground in this country, mainly owing to the anonymous work, entitled "Vestiges of Creation" — a volume it is impossible to read without wishing that the great ability of its author had been bestowed upon more authentic facts and sounder conclusions. A fair estimate of this doctrine, indeed, will lead us to see how much it owes to the intrinsic obscurity of the subject, and to the shelter of ambiguous language. We ridicule the *plastic power* of Cudworth; but its meaning is at least as valid as that of *appetencies, effort of internal sentiment,* and other similar phrases which have been since used to cover our ignorance of these elementary actions.

There is further cause to complain here of the covert use made of the term *Progressive Development,* for that which is virtually the doctrine of transmutation of species. These two phrases, and that also of *Successive Development,* require to be employed in every case with

The very general view I am taking of these subjects prevents my entering on this question, further than to express my belief that neither our present knowledge of facts, nor any principle of sound reason, will justify the admission of this doctrine. It is possible that the conceptions we attach to the term of *species* may require future modification, especially in the simpler and more rudimental forms of life. But at present every rule of philosophy calls upon us to recognise those strongly-marked distinctions which Nature has drawn by specific organisation and instincts; and to believe that the changes and varieties, superinduced upon them, are a part of that great scheme of mutual adaptation and limitation which we everywhere trace in the government of the world.

Reverting to our more immediate subject, we have first to notice the important distinction between animal and organic life, as regards the principle under discussion. Habits belong chiefly, if not exclusively, to the functions of animal life. Where they are perceived in those of

much exactness of definition, to avoid the many errors incident to their wrong application.

The question as to the existence in nature of *true species*, individual and permanent, has been more cogently revived of late by certain observations on hybrid animals and plants. These experiments require repetition, and admit in many ways of variation and extension. Some phrase may, perhaps, be hereafter substituted for *species*, better expressing the whole series of phenomena. Yet, well-defined as the word has been by Cuvier, De Candolle, and others; and admirably described as we find it by Lyell, in his " Elements of Geology," (37th chapter), we need hardly dismiss a term which has kept its place thus long in a science rapidly progressive; and which admits of ready qualification, should future progress require it.

organic life, it is under a more obscure and irregular form, and subject to a doubtful interpretation of their nature, from the intervention of the former even in those acts which seem most nearly organic in kind. In the functions of nutrition and excretion, as well as those of respiration and circulation, there is enough of the influence of animal life to justify the belief that it imparts something of its character to the vital actions with which it is blended.* The distinction then, just mentioned, must be considered a valid one; corresponding with the singular difference in the anatomy of the two systems, and illustrating well their other diversities. It is in the animal faculties, and thus associated with greater extent and complexity of nervous structure, that habits, rightly so understood, show themselves most distinctly, and have greatest sway over all the conditions of life. The familiar maxims on the subject are fully borne out by medical experience, and the practice of every physician abounds in curious illustrations of the fact.

Adopting here the division into bodily and mental habits, as that most natural in itself, we find many characteristic and striking examples of the former in the actions of the voluntary muscles, and especially in those co-ordinate actions already adverted to, which form so essential a part of the economy of life. In speaking, in walking, in the

---

* Bichat, pursuing into this subject his views of animal and organic life, strongly expresses their distinction as regards the dominion of habit: " Tout est modifié par l'habitude dans la vie animale ... Dans la vie organique nous verrons les phénomènes constamment soustraits à l'empire de l'habitude." This statement must be considered as liable to the qualification mentioned above.

thousand purposes for which we use the arms and hands, we unconsciously employ the most complex machinery, set in motion by the will, and altered or arrested by it; but while in action, governed and guided by habit alone. The series of consentient movements so produced is perfect enough in many cases to give the semblance of abstraction from all voluntary effort. That this ever really occurs we cannot, however, affirm; and the momentary changes required in many of these acts render the conception one very difficult to entertain. Even in cases where the mind appears most absent from the bodily phenomena, we must presume that the nervous power, acting on the muscular contractility, is constantly supplied while motion is going on. But with full admission of these doubtful points, the fact remains certain, that habit, due to frequent repetition, gives a co-ordinate action to groups of muscles, which they had not originally, and of which they may again be deprived by disease.

Or take other familiar instances in illustration, as when we balance the body to save it from falling, or make sudden movements to avert a blow, or adopt certain postures to relieve bodily pain. In none of these cases, could we predict a moment before what would be the actions fitted to fulfil these purposes. They are so instantaneous, and the machinery employed so entirely hidden from all common knowledge, that it is difficult to divest them of the semblance of instincts, brought suddenly into exercise. That they really belong to the class of habits is proved by the need of education and experience to give this power of instant adaptation; and by the perfection of their use being in exact proportion to its frequency.

Every part of this subject abounds in curious inferences. One remarkable result is the proof afforded of the limited nature of voluntary motions, compared with those of organic life. Not only do they come last in order, and require various education and effort to give them efficiency, but they soonest pass under the dominion of habit. The very exercise and repetition which renders them most perfect for use, removes them in a certain degree from that cognisance of consciousness which is essential to any just definition of the will. The most distinct acts of volition are those by which muscles are brought into modes of exercise altogether new. Of the combined and complex movements which form the common habits of these organs (for the action of a single muscle is a rare occurrence, if indeed it ever exist) more cannot be affirmed than that we will certain acts, which particular muscular combinations, wholly unknown to us in their details, are able to fulfil. If these combinations are incomplete, further trial and repetition, under suggestion of the will, are required to give the habits essential to more perfect use.

This conjunction of the voluntary power with actions tending to become automatic — performed, too, through organs which are shown to have an independent contractile power — brings us into contact with some of the most interesting questions in physiology. Experiment and observation, though they have done much, are not yet exhausted in reference to this subject. The minute examination, as far as may be possible, of the manner in which muscles are educated to particular acts and series of movements, is obviously a main source of further knowledge. The states of infancy and childhood, when this

natural education is in progress, might best furnish information, were it not that we have then no aid from the
mind, to expound its connexion with what is going on in
the material organs. Paralytic cases, while in course of
recovery of the voluntary power, may be studied with
greater advantage in this respect; as here, together with
the loss of voluntary power, there is usually also the partial loss of those habits of co-ordinate muscular action
which before existed. I have often obtained many curious
facts from the paralytic patient, thus occupied in re-
educating his muscles, and conscious himself of the effort
needed for this purpose, and of the means most successful
in effecting it.

The illustrations of Habit, as influencing the bodily
organs, might easily be multiplied by reference to the
many cases of anormal actions, arising from casual causes
of accident or disease, which by repetition become habitual
to the system, and often wholly uncontrollable by the
will. A familiar instance occurs in those irregular muscular actions, known under the name of *tricks;* where unmeaning movements take place automatically and without
the consciousness being awake to them. Other illustrations, again, might be drawn from functions in which the
mind and body are both concerned, of which sleep is a
marked example. But passing over these, I hasten to say
a few words regarding the habits of mental life more
exclusively, before closing this Chapter.

The term Habit, as applied to the recurrence in uniform
succession of particular states or acts of mind, in effect of re-

petition, is hardly less absolute in its meaning than when used to express the habitual mechanism of bodily movements. Apart even from all that belongs to natural temperament or propensities, we have the experience ever before us of mental habits created or destroyed by the varying incidents of life; and especially during the period of youth, when all impressions are more rapidly received, and more readily obliterated. We cannot wonder that much should have been written on this subject, seeing how momentous a part it bears in all the concerns of our intellectual and social life. Education does well in recognising this; for its most needful office is that of creating new habits of thought and action, or modifying those already created. On these matters it would be trite and unnecessary to dwell. Opinions are concurrent upon them; and the maxims in common use and drawn from common observation, though occasionally faulty or deficient, do yet mainly accord with the facts and suggestions derived from physiology. Yet, even with such general recognition, it may still be affirmed that practice is in the rear of principle on this point; and that the culture of mental habits, as distinguished from the mere acquisition of knowledge, is less explicitly regarded than it ought to be in our methods of education.

The formation of new habits, however, is not more important than is the control of those which are casually and often injuriously created, by the accidents of life, or by individual passions and propensities. These must be governed by the mind, that they may not gain dominion over it. They form an alien power in possession, which it needs strong efforts both of reason and resolution to expel.

To create and maintain "that vigour of mind which is able to contest the empire of habit," may be rightly denoted as the chief end of all moral discipline.*

Quitting this subject, however, as one more or less familiar to all, I must advert, before closing this Chapter, to another topic, which has only of late assumed its fit place as a branch of scientific inquiry, though of deep interest in every way to the history of man. I allude here to the influence of individual habits or peculiarities, whencesoever produced, in determining or modifying those of families, communities, and even races of mankind. In its first aspect, the assertion seems a bold one. But it is amply justified by observation, and by analogies derived from other parts of the animal world. The tendency of habits, whether bodily or mental — and even such as have been accidentally acquired — to become hereditary by pro-pagation, has been already noticed. What is true as to individuals and families, is not less so with regard to com-munities of men under similar physical and social condi-tions. Habits are gregarious in many ways, and to an extent beyond what would be deemed possible on a slight view of the subject. Contemplating their growth by here-ditary transmission, and especially in communities insu-lated by position and limited as to intermarriage, we obtain elements of the greatest importance towards the

---

* I quote these words from Locke, that I may have the occasion of stating how generally his precepts upon education are in accordance with the soundest views of modern physiology — a concurrence coming strongly in evidence of their truth. No system or rule of practice in education can safely be admitted, which does not associate itself with this part of science.

physical history of mankind in every country and age. Necessities, or even casualties of situation, long continued, may determine the habits of a people; and extend and perpetuate them as the permanent character of a race.

No adequate solution, indeed, can be given of the great problem of national diversities of character, without looking to the fact of habits, casual in their origin, becoming diffused and defined by hereditary descent. The proof of such diffusion within small circles is the interpretation of what must happen in the larger circles of the world,— with characters less explicit as the sphere becomes wider, but marked enough for sure evidence of the fact.* We cannot reject the conclusion that certain conditions of intellectual power and sensorial energy may thus become the property of particular races; together with physical peculiarities and other subordinate distinctions, all depending for their origin and development on the same common law. Nor, taking the extreme case, can we refuse to believe, that a single strong peculiarity of individual habit may be conveyed by this mysterious transmission through successive generations, blending itself in one degree or other with the existence of all, until finally lost through time and diffusion.

We are called upon here, indeed, to recognise another influence, concurring to the same result, and strongly attested by analogies from every part of organic life. This

---

* A curious illustration of the maintenance of particular family character through successive generations may be found in the history of some of the great families of ancient Rome. This observation, made by Niebuhr, will be recognised as true by all familiar with Roman history.

is the fact, that congenital deviations from the natural type (or *monstrosities*, as they are called in extreme cases,) do, under certain conditions, become hereditary and the foundation of subordinate varieties of the species. It is not easy to determine the amount of this influence, or what time and number of successions may render it wholly evanescent. But we cannot doubt that it forms one element in those great results which we have ascribed to the growth and transmission of habits through successive generations.

Scarcely can we exaggerate the interest of the questions and conclusions arising out of this inquiry. They will be seen to form an integral part of the physical and moral history of mankind, as spread in communities over the earth, and marked by especial diversities of outward lineament, character, and custom. The particular inquiries here relate to the conditions which favour such hereditary changes; the qualities of mind or body most liable to be so transmitted; the permanence of the changes produced; and the causes which limit or otherwise modify them. Much has been attained of late upon all these points of research; and the zeal and exactness with which every branch of Natural History, and especially that of Human Physiology, is now pursued, give certain assurance of the enlargement of our knowledge in this direction.*

* The physical history of mankind, in its larger sense, may be considered a new department of science. Almost all that has been done to give it a systematic form is comprised within the last half century; and the principal works of Dr. Prichard, the first great English labourer in the field, fall under this date. Geology — itself recent as a science — has of late rendered great aid to the history of

There is yet another part of this copious subject which I must notice, though unable to discuss it here. This is, the influence of Habit upon the course and treatment of disease. Much of what has already been said bears indirectly upon this topic, the importance of which no physician of experience can fail to recognise. The influence of habits can never safely be lost sight of in medical practice. Organs exercised so constantly in a given manner as to acquire, during health, some strong peculiarity or bias of action, are not merely liable to the intervention of certain disorders in effect of this; but, where the morbid cause is wholly alien to it, do still show its influence in the nature or degree of the symptoms produced. A particular function or faculty may become the subject of habits, so deeply impressed as to intercept the access of some morbid causes, while they aggravate the effect of others. The organs of animal life, and notably the brain and nervous system, furnish, as might be expected, the most frequent and explicit examples of this influence. But there are numerous cases, more obscure in kind, where it may still be recognised; both in the origin of morbid actions, and in the whole progress of the diseases consequent upon them.*

organic life in all its forms. To the writings of Sir C. Lyell, and to his own labours, together with those of other geologists, we are indebted for many and admirable illustrations of the connexion between animal life, and the successive conditions and changes of the surface of the globe.

* Must we not, for example, refer to some law or result of bodily habit, the comparative immunity from certain local causes of disease, which seems to be obtained by living long amidst them ? It is needful to admit, however, that this is an obscure matter, and requiring fuller verification by facts.

Whatever agency is thus strongly marked in creating or modifying disorder, must be of signal importance in all that concerns the treatment of it. And this, though hitherto perhaps inadequately regarded as a tenet of medical teaching or practice, is eminently true in reference to habits. The physician, while duly distinguishing between those which belong to natural temperament of mind or body, and such as have their origin in the casual incidents of life, will derive instruction and aid from both; and most especially in every thing that relates to the influence of mental affections on bodily disease. It would be beside my purpose to dwell further upon these topics here; but they well deserve to enter largely into every work on the principles and practice of medicine.

A general review of the topics treated of in the foregoing Chapter, will show how much is still wanting to their complete solution, or even to the exact discrimination of the questions they involve. Some of these questions indeed, as we have seen, are of a nature insuperable by any research we can hope to apply to them. But there are many others which form fitting matter of inquiry; and can hardly fail to repay it in the result. Modern science not merely works over a wider field, and with far greater exactness of observation and experiment, than heretofore; but it has acquired powers of combination and analysis transcending those of any former time, and still continually in progress towards higher perfection. The connexion of the different sciences is every day

CHAP. XI.

ON THE PRESENT STATE OF INQUIRY INTO THE
NERVOUS SYSTEM.

D'ALEMBERT has well designated the space which lies between geometry and metaphysics, " L'abîme des incerti-tudes et le théâtre des découvertes." A remarkable part of this wide intellectual domain is that occupied by the science of the nervous system; forming, in the present state of our knowledge, a sort of neutral ground between the sciences which deal with matter in its various forms, and those which have relation to the functions of animal life and mental existence. It is this common connexion with powers, which in their ultimate analysis by our reason are wholly incommensurate with each other, that gives to the subject its peculiar obscurity. Language here labours vainly to follow the suggestions of thought or consciousness; and the discussion has been endlessly perplexed by the efforts of philosophers to give phraseology to their doctrines, without any agreement as to the mean-ing of the terms employed.

The deep interest now felt in this branch of physiology, and the active and refined inquiry directed to it, may war-rant some observations on the subject, even though not adding to the facts already known. It is one of the cases in science where new conclusions and a nearer approach to

truth are rendered possible, simply by recasting the order
of these facts, and using them in new combinations.   In
the following remarks I shall touch only upon some parts
of this wide topic; not pretending to state in detail all
that has been accomplished of late years, but rather indicating the general results of the inquiry; and putting
much interrogatively, as best befitting what is still in
numerous respects so incomplete and obscure.   On certain
points (such, for instance, as the condition of *quantity*
in its application to the nervous power) I shall dwell
at greater length; from the consideration that they have
not hitherto been sufficiently examined.   On all parts of
the subject I shall seek to distinguish, as far as I am able,
between the several points which may yet be solved either
by anatomy or observation of the phenomena of life, and
those which a rational physiology will relinquish as beyond the scope of present attainment.*

Language, indeed, must not alone be charged with the
difficulties which belong to this research.   Our progress is
at every moment stopped; — on the one side, by the intricate and subtle organisation it is needful to decipher — on
the other, by thóse more insuperable bounds which, in the
very constitution of the human mind, seem destined to prevent too close a contemplation of its own workings; or

* Those who desire to learn the progress and actual state of knowledge on this subject will do well to refer to a series of most able
articles in the British and Foreign Medical Review; embracing its
relations to all other branches of physiology, as well as to the more
general principles of inductive science.   The physiological works of
Dr. Carpenter may be named with equal commendation, in reference
to this subject, and to all others of which they treat.

even of its manner of relation to the material instruments through which it acts. It may be that some men, by higher capacity of reason, whether invested in language or not — or by greater power of concentration, if this term better expresses the act of mind — do really approach nearer than others to the comprehension of these great functions of our nature. But every such difference is trifling in relation to the undiscovered and impassable space that lies beyond; and the highest attainment is that which can best define the boundary of research, and labour for truth and knowledge within it.

A question illustrating these remarks, and which stands indeed foremost in the inquiry, is that regarding the separate existence and attributes of the nervous power. Whatever censure has been thrown, justly or unjustly, upon this term, it is certain that we cannot dispense with some phrase equivalent to it, in reasoning on the phenomena of animal life. At every step we are obliged to admit the conception of the fact thus expressed; and however inadequate our present means to determine its nature, and relations to the mental and physical parts of our being, we can no more deny reality to such a power, than we can to the effects of which it is the obvious source. Other terms, — energy, agency, element, principle, and force — have, on the same grounds, been applied to denote it; all readily lending themselves to any relation with physical agents which may hereafter be ascertained; but liable in common to the preliminary objection of designating as one principle or element, that which we do not know to be really such. For the inquiry brings us at once to the most essential of the questions regarding the nervous power, viz., its unity:

R

— whether it be actually one and the same agent, producing diversity of effect from the manner of its transmission, or from the various fabric and vitality of the parts on which it acts; — or whether there are two or more powers coming under this common appellation as acting through nervous structure, but really different in nature, and thence producing different effects in the economy of life.

This question, to which I shall afterwards revert, becomes more definite as we proceed to specify the several functions appertaining to the nervous system, and especially those of the nerves of sensation and voluntary motion. Here the machinery obvious to examination is nearly or altogether alike; — it is everywhere blended for the purposes of mutual action and relation ; — yet are the functions themselves so utterly dissimilar to our comprehension, that we can in no way conceive the same physical agent, however modified, to be capable of fulfilling both. The opinion, early adopted by many physiologists, that the difference is simply that of the action being centripetal in the sensitive nerves, centrifugal in the motor, merely translates the difficulty into another form ; and is still less tenable since the distinctness of these two classes of nervous fibres has been fully demonstrated.

Nor do we remove it by regarding the nerves themselves merely as transmitters of power ; and, looking to one endowments of the ganglia as nervous centres, and to the independent contractility of the muscular fibre, respectively, as giving origin to these several actions. Such manner of viewing it is but a new expression of the difficulty ; — neither aiding our conception of the nature of

the power, nor of the manner in which it fulfils these dissimilar functions.

Other questions, analogous in kind and not less obscure,
suggest themselves in close connexion with those just
stated. Is it the same nervous power, merely altered in
the conditions of action, which is transmitted through the
nerves when a muscle is brought into voluntary use, as
when the same muscle is excited by mental emotions or
by reflex influence from some irritation of the sensory
nerves? Muscular contraction is produced by the will in
the one case — without the will, or even in opposition to
it, in the other. Must we suppose the force put into
action the same in both instances, the causes evolving it
being thus different?

The inquiry extends, and with equal difficulty of interpretation, to the nervous influence of organic life; using
this term to denote the power by which the several offices
of respiration, circulation, nutrition, and secretion, are
performed, without any direct action or intervention of
the senses or the will; though in such various and close
relation to these functions, that it seems as impossible to
dissever the respective operations as to understand their
dependence on a single source of power. — And yet further, in connexion with these organic functions, we are
required to recognise the direct influence upon them of all
mental emotions, even of the simple act of attention of
mind; — testified in every part of life, during sleep and
dreams, as well as in the waking state — connected with
some of the most remarkable sympathies of our nature —
and depending, we must suppose, upon relations of nervous
structure for all that concerns its direction to the several

organs of the body.   Further still, we have to look to the
nervous system as furnishing power for that *internuncial
office* (to use the phrase of John Hunter) by which the
connexions and mutual sympathies among different parts
of the body are maintained — not merely parts alike in
structure and function, but those also which fulfil totally
different purposes in the animal economy.   Must we suppose the nervous element, instrumental in these various
acts, to be identical with that which ministers to the functions of sensation and the will?   Or, if modified to meet
those widely different requirements, what are these modifications, and whence derived?

Such are some of the many problems as to this element
of nervous power or force, which meet us at the very
threshold of the inquiry.   Nor can we pause here amidst
these subordinate questions.   The course of human
thought, frequently urged forward by a speculative spirit,
has suggested the more abstruse form of inquiry : — whether there is not some superior and independent principle,
of which, however designated, the brain is the immediate
source and seat ; by which the animal functions are maintained and brought into relation with others, and unity
given to every part of the individual being ; — a principle
varying in power in different individuals, and forming
what has been termed the temperament of each;— varying
also in the same individual at different times, and, by its
excess or deficiency in the living organisation, becoming a
source of disorder to the functions both of body and mind?
Its definition, thus given, would call upon us to recognise
it in all the phenomena of health and disease ; from the
exuberant excitement of high bodily and mental vigour,

to the sudden collapse which threatens, or produces, instant death.   And we find terms appropriated to it, as well in the language of familiar use, as in that which has been current at all times in the schools of philosophy.

It is manifest that we are treading here on that obscure boundary between the mental and material functions, over which it has been the perpetual but fruitless aim of philosophy to pass.   It may be that the principle in question is not really a separate and single element of power, but merely a quality or degree of the other actions by which mind is connected with material organisation; — that we are not entitled to express more by it than a greater or less sensibility; a higher or lower degree of the voluntary power; or the varying strength of impressions made on the body by mental emotions.   This indeed is one part of that question, metaphysical more than physiological in its nature, which has perplexed reasoning men in every age, and been fruitful of dispute in proportion to its obscurity. We have powers before us for contemplation, which we cannot identify as the properties of any physical agents, nor interpret by any analogy beyond their own action; and which, while giving unity to many separate organs and functions, seem to be derived from, and supported by, the combination of these functions themselves.   On the other side we must regard them as indissolubly blended with the great separate unity of the mind and will; a relation which, from the very conditions of the inquiry, must ever remain a closed question to the present comprehension of man.*

* These observations apply to the notion held by some authors of the existence of another sense, needful to establish a community of

On many of these points it is expedient for the highest interests of science, that inquiry should not, by any mere artifices of language, be pressed beyond this boundary. Though insusceptible of strict definition, it is certain and obvious as a general limit, and becomes more so as our knowledge increases in exactness. The precaution suggested by one of the wisest of the ancients, Το γινωσκειν τινων δεἰ ζητειν αποδειξιν, καὶ τινων ου δεὶ, is applicable to every age of philosophy. Within this boundary, indeed, there is space enough for the utmost zeal of research; and it is enlarged, rather than narrowed, by the abandonment of all abstractions which are not absolutely requisite to classify the phenomena observed.

These remarks directly apply to the much-debated question of a Vital Principle; — a term more familiar to common use, but which, in strict definition, can hardly be detached from the power we have just had under consideration. Expressing an agency independent of organisation, and itself capable of organising and giving life, it has found its way into every part of physiology and general philosophy; and, even where rejected by men of acute understanding, is still often seen to lurk in their writings, under some less palpable form of expression. In reasoning, for example, on the active principle of animal organisation — that which operates in the original evolution and unceasing maintenance of the animal frame — some modern physiologists have almost given separate existence to this, as the *primum movens* of the system; therein approaching

feeling and consciousness in all parts of the body; the *Gemeingefühl* or *Selbstgefühl* of German physiologists.

to the theory of Stahl and early writers; and still more closely to the doctrine of which we are speaking, in one or other of the forms it has assumed.* For even under what seems a simple phraseology we find much latitude of definition, and a tendency to apply the term of Vital Principle either to mental or material phenomena, according to the genius or opinions of the particular author.

Upon this subject, however, I do not speak at greater length, having nothing to add to what has been so ably written upon it of late years. To suppose the existence of a principle of life, independent of the organs and functions of living bodies, and superadded to give activity to them, would seem, in the present state of our knowledge, the substitution of a mere phrase for the reality of facts. We gain from it no explanation of the vital actions and affinities, the relations of which are the proper objects of study; nor even of the phenomena of generation, and of propagation by simple division in some of the lower animals, which seem most to authorise the conclusion; — but

---

* In describing the principle of organisation (the *nisus formativus* of early writers), the German physiologists have availed themselves of the richness and redundance of their language to give a more copious and distinct expression of these powers than any we have ventured to adopt. No other modern language could furnish such phrases as " *Die bewustloss wirkende zweckmässige Thatigteit.*" — " *Die nach vernunftigen Gesetzen wirkende organizirende Kraft,*" &c., which we find in the writings of Müller, and which appear to give more of individuality and independence to this power than is usually recognised at the present day. His discussion of the question of identity, or other relation, of the mental principle (*Das Psychische Princip*) to that of life, is a striking specimen of the acuteness of this eminent physiologist.

rather impose injurious limits on all other parts of the
inquiry which are fairly open to research. We interpose
a separate agent, (for in no other sense can the doctrine of
a vital principle, thus independent, be understood), when
all that is warranted to our understanding is the assumption of existing and active laws.

I have dwelt longer on these topics, as illustrating the
peculiar difficulties of the subject, and the manner in which
they both direct and limit the course of all research into
the nervous system. Of the various modes of conducting
this inquiry, the simplest would seem to be that of considering—first, the complex material organisation by which
nervous power is generated, and through which it is transmitted in fulfilment of its offices ;—secondly, the relations
subsisting between different portions of that nervous structure and the particular functions of animal and organic
life ;—and thirdly, the element of nervous power itself;
hitherto defined to us only by its various and wonderful
effects, and so far inaccessible, as we have seen, to physical
research, that we cannot even affirm its absolute unity of
nature ; yet affording certain determinate conclusions and
promising more to future inquiry. To this outline I shall
chiefly adhere in further discussing the subject; — limiting
myself, in accordance with the general plan of the volume,
to those points especially which regard the nervous system
as it is developed in man.

Here, indeed, it is that we find the highest example of
this organisation and of the functions depending on it,
which come within our present knowledge or conception.
From the simple and elementary forms of nervous matter
which the microscope has detected in some of the Radiata,

there is a progressive development of this system as we
ascend in the scale of the animal creation — in some cases
by the addition of new organs, in others by the modification of anterior types; — every such stage of progress
having specific relation to the uses and necessities of the
forms of animal life in which it is manifested.   In the Vertebrate animals we first find those cerebral lobes and cerebellum, forming the true brain.   In the Mammalia this
organisation is greatly advanced.   In Man it reaches its
highest development, and largest proportion to the rest of
the nervous system.   The general relation thus maintained
throughout between the degree of nervous development
and the perfection of the animal functions, incontestibly
establishes this connexion.   And in so doing it places before the mind a certain conception of the manner in which
functions and endowments, yet higher than those of man,
might be associated with organised structure, and thus
brought into various and active relation with the external
world.   Science leads us by legitimate steps to the entrance
of this avenue, and affords a glimpse of what may lie
beyond.   But it leaves us at this point; nor can analogy
guide us further to any certain or profitable result.*

The application of anatomy to the brain and nerves has
the double object of disclosing the intimate structure of
nervous matter itself under its different forms, and of indi-

---

* Adopting it as an inference from the whole course of nature in
the animal creation, Locke strongly expresses his opinion on this subject.
" That there should be more species of intelligent creatures above us,
than there are of visible or material below us, is probable to me from
hence, that in all the corporeal world we see no chasms or gaps."

cating its manner of distribution and connexion, as masses, trunks, or branches, throughout the various parts of the body. The latter direction of research is at present the most important to physiology; seeing the difficulty of drawing any plausible conclusion even from the most minute examination of nervous structure.* This examination begun by Ehrenberg with more refined use of the microscope than heretofore — and ably and indefatigably pursued by other physiologists — has, it is true, disclosed many very curious facts; which, though yet fruitless of inference, may hereafter be of avail in explaining some of the obscure phenomena of the nervous system. Such are especially — the distinction between the tissue of globular cells, enveloped in blood vessels, which constitutes the proper cineritious or ganglionic structure, and the tubular or gelatinous filaments forming the true nervous fibres — the structure of the cylindrical nerve-tube, covered by a membranous neurilema, and containing a soft viscous matter, more fluid in the brain than the nerves, continuous through each nerve, and obviously forming an essential part of its economy—the absolute distinctness and isolation of each primitive nervous fibre throughout its whole course—the varying size of these tubular fibres in different parts of the cerebral and nervous organisation—the close intertexture of blood-vessels with neurine, wherever the

---

* Professor Alison in his Physiology, describes the nervous system as "living and growing within an animal, as a parasitic plant does within a vegetable;" — an analogy that may seem at first somewhat vague, but which on reflection will be found to afford several suggestions of great interest in this part of physiology.

latter exists—and the identity of structure, as far as examination can go, of the sentient and motor nerves.*

Many subordinate results might be added to these; together with some of equal importance, but not yet sufficiently confirmed.   Though attention has been actively directed to the question, there is still much doubt as to the manner of origin of the nervous fibres, whether afferent or efferent in function; and also as to their mode of termination on the sentient surfaces and in the muscular tissue, whether by anastamosis of loops and network, or by separate extremities.   A further controversy exists, which has evoked all the powers of the microscope, as to the nature of the nervous fibres belonging to the great Sympathetic system;—in what respects of size, colour, and texture they differ from the cerebral and spinal nerves. Nor is the manner of connexion yet fully determined between the fibrous tissue of the white or medullary portion of the brain, and the granular or globular texture of the cineritious part; a point of relation which we must necessarily regard as one of the most important in the whole nervous system.

Interesting though these results are as detached facts, it

---

* Among the numerous Continental physiologists who have recently and successfully prosecuted this research into the minute anatomy of the brain and nerves, the names of Müller, Valentin, Remak, Foville, Burdach, Schwann, and Kölliker, may especially be mentioned.   This particular branch of the inquiry has been somewhat less actively pursued in England; but taking the whole subject of the nervous system, our anatomists and physiologists have fully maintained the reputation of English science by their zeal and success.   And it would be easy to name many eminent men now amongst us, whose labours are laying the foundation of further discovery in this path of pursuit.

will be seen that they afford no certain clue to the
elementary actions and combinations occurring in the
nervous system. Nor can it even be shown that the parts
thus described are really the ultimate elements of nervous
structure. In no part, indeed, of physical science are we
able to affirm that our analysis has yet reached these
ultimate parts (the μεγεθη αδιαιρετα) of the bodies with
which we are dealing. Least of all is this likely to happen as regards the material of the nervous substance; the
functions of which are so far removed from all that falls
within the cognisance of the senses, or our common understanding of physical actions. The most important, and
perhaps the most assured inference we obtain from the
minute anatomy just described, is, the distinction between
the offices of the cineritious parts of the brain, spinal marrow, and ganglia; and of the white, or true nervous, portion of these organs and of the nerves generally throughout the body. The peculiar diversity of structure in these
two tissues affords much reason for concluding that the
agent of nervous power, however designated, is evolved by
the former; while by the latter it is variously distributed
and applied to the manifold uses or necessities of animal
existence.* Yet even here it will be seen how closely our

---

* Of the several opinions propounded as to the origin of the nervous power, that stated above is certainly best sanctioned by observation. The complex and highly vascular structure of the cineritious
part (as determined by the microscope and by the fine injections of
Dr. Arnold of Zurich) is strikingly contrasted with the straight
cylindrical fibres, chiefly composing the medullary portion. And this
difference, while indicating different offices, strongly presses the conclusion that the latter is the conducting medium to the power generated in the former.

knowledge is limited to the expression of this presumed fact; and that we obtain no ulterior inference, either as to the nature of this power, or the conditions and changes which make it capable of fulfilling functions so various and dissimilar in the economy of life. If these results of minute anatomy are ever associated with more exact knowledge, it will probably happen rather from the growth of science without, than from any internal evidence they can themselves afford.

The same remarks will apply to the facts derived from the chemical examination of neurine or nervous matter. Of the small proportion of solid ingredients, the greater part is albuminous or fatty substance, associated with two organic acids, — the sole peculiarity of the analysis being the extraordinary quantity of phosphorus present, in the proportion sometimes of nearly one-twentieth of the whole solid matter.   That this elementary body (as we are obliged yet to consider it) is essential to the constitution of nervous substance cannot be doubted.   But the fact is hitherto a fruitless one in our hands; nor can we carry even conjecture one step beyond it.

One of the most important facts derived from these researches is that of the intimate connexion of the nervous and vascular systems, — the close and constant intertexture of nerves and blood-vessels throughout every part of the body; and especially in those organs whence the nerves originate and in the sentient surfaces over which they are diffused. In saying that this connexion is maintained through the capillary arteries, we express, in reality, the most active and energetic form which such relations can assume. The arterial trunk is but the conduit for blood. All the more important offices of this great moving agent of life are performed through a mechanism of parts, vascular or interstitial, so exquisitely minute and complex that our finest instruments can hardly find access to the spaces within which they are included.* And, without reference to certain points in this subtle organisation, concerning which there is yet dispute, whenever we see these capillary vessels closely and uniformly blended with other organs, we may deem it certain that important functions are involved, common and essential to the design of both.

What this obvious structural connexion of the nerves and blood-vessels would alone suffice to prove is confirmed by other more general considerations. We cannot designate a single part in the whole economy of animal life in which we do not find these two great powers conjointly concerned ; — their co-operation so essential that no single function can be perfectly performed without it. The blood and the nervous force, as far as we know, are the only agents which actually pervade the body throughout ;

* "What the immensity of creation is to the astronomer or geologist, such are these infinitely small dimensions of matter in space to the physiologist. Presuming, or knowing, that all organisation, however minute, such as the many thousand lenses which compose an insect's eye, must be due to the agency of distinct vessels — circulating, secreting, and absorbing — we have some vague measure of that exquisite minuteness of fabric and formative action, upon which life in its several parts essentially depends."

I venture to quote this from a Chapter in my former work (Chap. xxx. On Disturbed Balance of Circulation) with the view of referring at the same time to a more detailed discussion which will be found there, on this very important subject of the connexion of the nervous and circulating systems.

the connexion of the machinery by which they are conveyed becoming closer, as we have seen, in proportion as
we get nearer to the ultimate limits of observation.   Besides those results of their co-operation which have regard
to the numerous other objects and phenomena of life, we
cannot doubt the existence of a reciprocal action upon
each other, necessary to the maintenance and completeness of their respective powers.   It is impossible, for
obvious reasons, to define the nature of this reciprocity, or
to determine in which agent the power was first evoked.
We cannot adopt the phrase of *innervation* of the blood —
nor even that of its *vitality,* sanctioned by the eminent
name of John Hunter — under any conception distinct
enough to warrant further inferences from them.   Nor
can we follow with any clear understanding the notion of
the nervous element as evolved by the agency of the blood ;
or as actually *derived from* the blood, and depending for
its maintenance and energy on the conditions of this fluid.
Yet we can hardly doubt that mutual actions and relations
of some such nature do really exist.   Evidence to this
effect is furnished, directly or indirectly, by all the natural
phenomena of health, and even more remarkably by the
results of disorder and disease.   The whole inquiry is of
singular importance to the physiology of animal life ; and,
though beset with many difficulties, can hardly fail to
yield much that is valuable to future investigation.

Passing now from this more minute anatomy to the
general view of the structure, distribution, and connexion
of the several parts forming the nervous system, we find
it almost as difficult to classify, as to enumerate, the facts
derived from the industry and refinement of modern re-

search. One marked scheme of division, indeed, offers itself, which cannot rightly be disregarded; that, namely, into the Cerebral hemispheres and Cerebellum—the system of the Cerebro-spinal axis—and that of the great Sympathetic nerve. While following this outline generally, it is needful, at the same time, to keep in constant view the functions of the several parts, as far as they are yet ascertained; illustrations drawn from this source being necessary to the understanding even of the simplest facts which anatomy lays before us. In no branch of medical science, indeed, is the connexion closer between dissection and experimental physiology. The latter becomes absolutely essential to the exposition of parts which are so inter-blended and bound together, that the outward aspect gives no sort of explanation of their endowments, and experiment is required to interpret relations seemingly the most obvious to the eye. Our knowledge of the symmetrical nerves of the spine might be termed barren, until the great discovery of Sir C. Bell, of the separate functions of the anterior and posterior roots, not merely determined the especial offices of these parts, but indicated further the right mode of research as applied to other analogous structures. It is here also, in the connected examination of structure and functions, that Comparative Anatomy and Comparative Physiology are of greatest avail; illustrating, by successive addition of parts and endowments, the mutual relations of all.

The instance just quoted forms a part of what must be considered one of the greatest attainments in the physiology of the nervous system; viz., the more exact definition of the structure and offices of the cerebro-spinal axis; in its relation, on the one side, to involuntary or instinctive actions; on the other, to the sensations and volitions which connect the mind with the material organisation around it. The results recently obtained have removed errors obscuring all former views on this subject; and the minute dissections which have shown, not only the distinctions of different parts of the spinal cord, but also a continuous structure of nervous fibres, extending severally from them, through the medulla oblongata, to the sensory ganglia; and thence brought into relation, by a new system of commissures or nervous connexions, with the cerebral hemispheres — these dissections illustrate (though they cannot explain) the combinations of mental and automatic acts which may well be reckoned among the most singular phenomena of animal life.

It is indeed through this important portion of the nervous system, the cerebro-spinal axis, (including the medulla spinalis, medulla oblongata, and the sensorial ganglia within the cranium), that we have acquired our most valuable knowledge in this part of physiology. Its automatic character, and independence of the cerebral lobes and cerebellum, is shown by the maintenance of its functions for a considerable time, even where these organs are absent from original defect or from subsequent removal. Yet here it is that we find those connexions established of feeling and motion, which are essential to the very definition of animal existence; — here, also, that we detect, either by observation or inference, the instrumental part of the numerous sympathies of mind and body which belong more especially to man. The most remarkable among these sympathies (and even involving, as we have

s

seen, the question of the unity of the nervous power), are those which depend on the relations of nerves of different endowments; — the excitement of motion in one part by sensation in another; or, conversely, of sensation by motion; the connexion of both with the peculiar nervous functions of organic life; and the relation of all to the acts and emotions of mind.

The most important step which has been made in this part of physiology is the determination of those sympathetic or reflex actions between the sentient and motor nerves which occur directly through the medulla spinalis, without intervention of the brain. The discovery of these relations, which we owe to the labours of Dr. Marshall Hall, has greatly extended and better defined our knowledge of the whole economy of the nervous system, and has proved of singular value to every part of pathology, as well as in explanation of the natural functions of the body.* It establishes, as the result of observation and experiment, a simply automatic part of this system, with which the perceptions and volitions of the mind are only indirectly concerned, and which has within itself the instruments of sensibility and motion; producing actions antecedent, as it seems, to all others in time; and to which the true cerebral and intellectual functions are added gradually, blending with and modifying, but never

---

* The importance of Dr. M. Hall's researches cannot be duly estimated without regarding them in their relation to pathology. They illustrate (as he has himself very successfully indicated in his writings) many diseases and morbid states of the nervous system, which had before been imperfectly understood, or often wholly misinterpreted as to their origin and progress.

superseding them.   The manner of connexion of these automatic impressions and motions with the various phenomena of instinct has been fully considered in the last Chapter.   I do not recur to it here further than by repeating, that it is the instrumentality only of instinctive action which is thus partially explained; and that we gain no clue thereby to the real nature of these phenomena, as connected with material organisation.

Though so much has been done towards the anatomy of the spinal cord, several points are yet imperfectly solved. Some ambiguity still exists as to the especial offices of the columns composing it, and also as to the question whether there is in any part of its structure an arrangement by transverse segments, corresponding with the particular endowments of each portion.   Much is to be learnt as to the commissures or decussations between the portions of the cord.   And further, it yet remains to be proved, whether there is any especial structure belonging to the reflex actions performed through the cord and medulla oblongata, independently of the brain and cerebral nerves ; — a peculiar spinal system, on the excitor and motor nerves of which depend the mechanism of respiration, the ingestion and egestion of aliment, and the actions generally of the orifices and sphincters throughout the body.   Research has been already directed to this point, the importance of which to the whole theory of organic life is the best security for its eventual determination. *

---

* I allude here to the able treatise of Mr. Grainger, in confirmation of Dr. Marshall Hall's opinions ; in which he offers evidence of the anatomical distinctness of the nerves concerned in reflex action.

The distinctive term of Medulla Oblongata, in describing a part of the great nervous axis of the body, is, perhaps, unnecessary; inasmuch as it is essentially a prolongation of the spinal cord upwards into the sensory ganglia of the cranium. The automatic functions, indeed, which have their especial origin in this part, are of a nature absolutely essential to animal life. Respiration, and the various acts which belong to the deglutition of food, though subject to some voluntary influence, yet are effectively and independently maintained by the reflex actions occurring here; and by the many complex and peculiar connexions of the nerves which minister to these great functions. The phenomena, so automatically associated in these parts, abound in curious and unexpected facts. Thus in the experiments of Flourens, if admitted as free from ambiguity, we obtain evidence that the acts belonging to the mechanism of respiration have their origin in a segment of the medulla oblongata, which he estimates at not more than a line in thickness.* While from the recent researches of M. Bernard we derive the still

This evidence is strengthened by Dr. Carpenter's examination of what is analogous in the nervous system of the Invertebrata; but it still falls short of entire proof.

* These experiments of M. Flourens, reported to the French Academy at the close of 1851, were made in repetition of his former researches on the same subject. They define more exactly what he calls the "*Point premier moteur de mécanisme respiratoire;*" where an injury inflicted, or an incision insulating this point from the spinal marrow above, produces instant suspension of the respiratory functions, and death. "La quantité de substance blessée ou isolée n'est pas plus grosse que la tète d'un épingle. C'est donc de l'integrité d'un point si petit, que depend la vie du systeme nerveux, la vie de l'animal, en un mot, la vie."

more singular fact, that an injury done to a certain part of this nervous tract produces an immediate secretion of sugar from the kidneys.   Phenomena like these show how much is wanting to our full comprehension of the attributes of the nervous system ; and above all, how little we can conceive that wonderful power which thus localises its action in particular portions of the material machinery of life.

In alluding to the sensory ganglia as the remaining portion of the cerebro-spinal axis, and to the whole system of cerebral nerves, I must limit myself to the mere mention of those refined and beautiful researches by which it has been sought to determine the relations and offices of these several parts.   That various points still remain undecided will not excite the wonder of any one who is aware of the singular complexities of structure and distribution in this part of the nervous system ; and of those peculiar obstacles to experiment, which even make it difficult, in some cases, to determine whether a nerve is one of sensation or motion. The extent to which all such difficulties have been overcome (and especially in the instances of the fifth pair of nerves, the par vagum, the accessory nerve, &c.), is the best proof of the zeal and ability given to the inquiry. Here indeed, as in every other department of physical science, we possess not solely a more just definition of the objects than heretofore, but methods of research far more exact, and instruments both of observation and experiment infinitely excelling those of any former time.*   The

* Much might be said, did it come within our subject, upon the remarkable advancement, as to all these points, in the progress of physical science during the last hundred years, and most conspicuously

results of the labours so conducted I cannot give here, having already explained the limitation of this Chapter to a general view of the knowledge hitherto obtained on the subject, and to an indication of those points most reasonably open to further inquiry.

Omitting, then, these details, we come at once to that greatest member of the nervous system, the Cerebral Hemispheres; a part which, from its magnitude, peculiarities of structure, and progressive development from the lower vertebral animals up to man, is manifestly of peculiar importance to the higher faculties of our being. Our present state of knowledge regarding the brain involves the same questions we have seen to apply to other parts of the nervous system, — multiplied in number and difficulty by that closer involution of parts which has suggested the description of it as a group of ganglia—and by the nearer approach to the mental functions, if a phrase involving the notion of space be admissible, for what we cannot conceive to have any common or congruous quality with it. When we get beyond the apparent connexions and terminations (the latter term itself ambiguous) of the sensory and motor nerves prolonged from the spinal columns, the anatomy of the hemispheres affords little more than

---

within the last half century. The better definition of the principles and methods of inquiry has contributed to the exactness of results even more than the perfection of the instruments and means employed. La Place well denotes the value of *Methods*, as a foundation of all such researches: — " La connaissance *de la Methode* qui a guidé l'homme de génie, n'est pas moins utile au progrés de la science, et même à sa propre gloire, que ses decouvertes."

certain uniform appearances, variously arranged by different observers; and physiology is confined to insulated
facts, drawn chiefly from pathology, or from comparative
anatomy and experiments on living animals. All these
classes of facts have been greatly extended, and many
remarkable presumptions derived from them. Nevertheless, examining fairly into the subject, it will be seen how
few are the conclusions which can be recorded as final
and complete. Pathological observations, however great
their ultimate value, have hitherto, by their discordance,
rather perplexed than illustrated the inquiry ; and the
results of actual experiments so partially concur with
these, and with each other, that almost every inference
requires to be verified by further research.

The phenomena of the brain in its healthy state, the
particular effects of lesion or disease, the congenital deficiencies of its structure in idiots, and the results of experiments made upon it, have seemed to some physiologists
to warrant the phrase of " the seat of intellectual functions," as applied to the cerebral hemispheres. A better
expression, because more consistent with our knowledge,
is, that the organisation of these parts so ministers to
certain mental faculties and conditions, that any deficiency
or injury of structure impairs in some proportionate
degree the functions thus connected. For reasons already
given, it is very important in this inquiry to restrict
language to the simple denotation of facts. The complex
nature of these faculties, — needfully separated for description, yet indicated as a unity to our consciousness, —
is itself sufficient cause for the utmost use of caution in
all the conclusions we derive from them.

The most assured of these conclusions is probably that which regards the cerebral hemispheres as serving especially to the functions of memory and association, in the simplest understanding of the terms. To this subject I have alluded in a former Chapter; stating the reasons — and especially those derived from the observed effects of injury or disease — which make it likely that these faculties (including the recollective power) are more closely related to material organisation than any other attributes of mind.* The very phrase of *Memoria Technica*, and the methods and artifices included under it, are a familiar testimony to the same effect. Seeing the pre-eminence of these faculties in man, the large part of life they fill, and their necessity to other intellectual functions, we might naturally expect some principal and conspicuous part of the brain to appertain to their exercise. But admitting the Cerebrum to fulfil this condition, we are unable to carry our conclusions beyond; or to form any conception of the manner in which these functions are actually performed. Further than this, we have every assurance that other offices also belong to this great central organ, — and in particular that of the establishment of connexion between the several parts of the nervous system; and between each part and that *Sensorium Commune* which is concerned in the functions of all; — a name I purposely use, though very ambiguous in its meaning, to indicate once more the difficulty of finding clear terms for the ex-

* See Chap. VII., "On the Memory as affected by Age and Disease." Some physiologists have supposed the faculties of speech and language to be especially associated with the anterior lobes of the cerebrum; but the evidence is hardly sufficient for this deduction.

pression of that unity, of which our consciousness is unceasingly informing us.

For here, again, we find ourselves involved in those speculations regarding the connexion of the mind itself, and its higher faculties, with material organisation, which have been the subject of controversies in every age of philosophy. I have already spoken on this topic (p. 171.), and I refrain from recurring to it, not merely as one exhausted in argument, but believing the relation to be one wholly inapproachable by human reason. I will merely remark, in correction of a common misapprehension on the subject, that the further we proceed in unravelling the brain as a collection of nervous fibres, condensed into separate organs for the establishment of their several functions and relations, the more in fact do we detach the mind itself from all material organisation. By showing the general similarity of the minute cerebral tissue to those other portions of the nervous structure which conduct sensations or volitions, and minister to automatic acts — functions all subordinate to the mental principle — we disconnect the latter with any matter obvious to our senses or most refined instruments of research. And while allowing the influence of every part of the brain upon it, and of some parts more than others, we still more directly annul the assumption that these material functions are in themselves acts or conditions of mind. It may be requisite for sensation, that impressions should be transmitted through certain series of nerves to the Cerebrum; but this gives no local tenement to the sentient principle, nor explains in any way its relation to the matter which is thus instrumental for its uses.

I allude especially to these points, because it is a frequent error, both of those who indulge in and those who dread and deprecate such speculations, to suppose that in proving these particular connexions we tend to identify the actions of matter with the operations of mind. Were research a hundredfold more minute and certain in its results, the separation of the two would remain to all comprehension exactly what it now is. But, in truth, both anatomy and physiology are still engaged in settling points of structure far below those of the ultimate organisation of the brain. Many of the appearances in ordinary dissection are probably owing, not to the true nervous matter, but to the membranous coverings which every where accompany and invest it. Even those microscopic observations which show the tubular structure of the medullary fibres, leave all uncertain as to the peculiar matter existing within. Chemistry, as we have seen, gives no indications on which to found a single inference; and the conclusions from pathology are rendered vague and insufficient by dealing only with the grosser parts of structure and connexion. These difficulties are capable of being overcome up to a certain point. But such as attach directly to the relations between organised structure and the mind are insuperable in their nature; and we may best serve the interests of science by leaving them aside from the direction of our pursuit.

There are, however, certain points of more general relation here, which have reasonably been made the subjects of active inquiry. Such are, the relative size and proportions of these organs to the different degrees of intelligence in the scale of animal life. The methods of research on these subjects are obviously of approximation only; but the results are so far concurrent as fully to justify the inferences drawn from them. Whether we take the facial angle of Cooper, — or the comparative area of sections of the cranium and face, as proposed by Cuvier,— or the proportionate size of the cerebrum to the medulla oblongata and spinal cord in the different classes of vertebrate animals,—equally do we see the growth of these great cerebral organs in approaching towards man, and the high ratio they bear in him towards those of mere sentient or organic life. The conclusions hence obtained are of high interest to all our views of animal existence, as spread over the globe we inhabit.

The doctrines of phrenology are closely associated with this part of the subject; but having examined them in a preceding Chapter, I do not recur to the topic here. Another curious question, (also discussed before,) is that of the condition of the brain as a double organ — the inferences suggested by the fact of unity of action and result from this doubleness of parts—-and the possible or certain effects of differences of the two sides, however produced, or of morbid changes in the commissures connecting them. Without repeating the argument, I may advert once more to the singular importance of these connecting structures, whatever form they assume. We cannot venture further to define their office than as blending double and similar parts into single and consentaneous action. But limiting our view to this point, we must regard the integrity of their functions as essential to the healthy condition of the brain; and their morbid changes, as far as dissection can discover them, become of great interest in the history of various cerebral and mental disorders.

No stronger proof can be given of the deficiencies in our actual knowledge of the brain than the uncertainty still existing as to the true offices of the Cerebellum. From its size, position, connexions, and peculiar structure, we cannot doubt that it fulfils purposes essential to the higher conditions of animal life. Its association with the Cerebrum is so intimate (whatever the exact nature of this) that where the latter does not exist, the Cerebellum is always found to be wanting. We may presume with certainty that it is concerned in the origin or direction of some particular actions of the nervous power; but the contradictory opinions or confessed ignorance of physiologists on the subject, leave this remarkable question still open to future discovery. The opinion adopted by Gall and his followers, that it is the organ of sexual impulse, is insufficiently attested by facts. There is more reason, from the experiments of the Continental physiologists, to suppose that it is concerned in combining and regulating the co-ordinate muscular movements throughout the body. But there is so much that is vague in this definition of object, and the experiments themselves are often so ambiguous, that we must needs acquiesce in the avowal I have just stated.*

---

* The experiments of Flourens and Hertwig, if deficient in complete proof of the functions of the Cerebellum, are at least incompatible with the phrenological view of this organ. In illustration of the doubts still hanging over this question, I could mention one or two cases of which I have notes, where, though the want of proper direction of the movements of the body was a conspicuous symptom, the

The whole complex apparatus of the Sympathetic Nerves and its ganglia — forming that division of the nervous system which appertains chiefly to the functions of organic life — is another part of what we must still consider the *terra incognita* in this great domain of physiological inquiry. Its anatomy is in every point very intricate and obscure ; and its physiological relations must be put interrogatively even for the organs and functions which appear to have closest dependence upon them. Closely associated though the Sympathetic system is with the great functions of nutrition and secretion, it has been reasonably doubted, upon the analogies of vegetable life, whether it is essential to these simple vital acts.   The manner of connexion of this system with the cerebro-spinal presents a long series of unresolved questions ; and the experiments of Dr. W. Philip and others, while deciding certain points, have added to the number remaining for solution.   The nature and offices of the ganglia appended to it — whether generating, or merely modifying and directing the passage of power from the greater nervous centres — are known to us but by presumption, and this hitherto too vague to be recorded as matter of science. The intimate connexion of the Sympathetic nerves with the vascular system throughout — their probable agency in the effects of mental emotions upon the vital organs — and their general relation to the irritability of the body —

---

post mortem examination showed no morbid changes in the cerebellum.   It must be admitted, however, that our common dissections in diseases of the brain, though much improved, are still not exact enough for the conclusions we seek to draw from them.

are all points of similar and equal interest to physiology, but not less obscure in every circumstance of present proof.*

From this review of what is known, and what not yet known, of the anatomy and functions of the nervous system, we reach at once the very important question as to the existence and properties of a physical agent, operating through the brain and nerves as the instrument of the several offices they fulfil. This question is one wholly separate from the metaphysical speculations to which I have lately alluded; and may be entertained (whatever the ultimate success of the research) as legitimately as any other inquiry in science. It has, in truth, been much and variously discussed; by some only as a vague hypothesis, having its foundation chiefly in the phraseology applied to it — by other and more eminent authors, experimentally, and as a well-defined object of research. I have already alluded to the question in the early part of this Chapter; and to the various terms employed to express this power or force of which we are speaking. Its consideration may now be more advantageously resumed, in sequel to our review of the functions of the nervous system, and of what has been done by anatomy and physiology in relation to this subject.

We are compelled, indeed, to be cautious as to language

* In Chap. II. of this volume I had occasion to allude to certain of these doubtful questions, in reference to the subject then before me; viz., the Influence of Mental Attention on the Bodily Organs. We have strong presumptive reasons for looking to the nerves of the Sympathetic system as concerned in some of these effects.

here ; since even at the threshold of the inquiry we are met by the question, whether that which we term nervous power depends on a separate physical agent or element, formed or evolved within the body, and acting through the peculiar organisation of the nervous system? — or whether, in the absence of strict demonstration, we must confine our expressions to that of simple power or force, without denoting whence this is derived, or supposing any new material element to be concerned in the phenomena depending on it? It is the same question, and suggested by similar considerations, as that-recently applied to the other imponderable principles, light, heat, electricity, and chemical force; testifying in this the rigour of modern science in all its methods and deductions; and showing, at the same time, the higher principles and relations which are now submitted to inquiry. That certain singular relations of analogy, if not of more intimate kind, do subsist between the nervous power and one or more of the great forces just named, cannot be doubted. Many of the questions of greatest difficulty are the same in each case ; and though it may seem in electrical actions (taking these as the example, and using the term in its largest sense) that the effects of a material agent are much more certain and obvious to sense; yet, strictly analysed, we find these phenomena not to express more than we can legitimately assign as the attributes and manner of action of the true nervous power.

The most philosophical, as well as convenient method of illustrating the latter, is indeed in principle the same as that we apply to the investigation of the laws of electricity, magnetism, &c.; as will, I think, appear in the remarks I shall have to make on this curious subject. Though we cannot prove by demonstration to the senses, or actual experiment, that there exists a distinct material element in what we term nervous power; yet there are so many properties which we cannot otherwise conceive or describe than as *functions of matter in motion,* that we seem justified in adopting some such principle as the basis of inquiry.* The existence, and the various and diffused action of this element throughout the body, is indeed demonstrated in the same sense, and almost in the same way, as that of the circulation of the blood. We have every reason to suppose certain organs appropriated to its production or evolution; others to its modification or the direction of its passage to different parts. The remarkable arrangement of nerves in the body, whether single, or collected into central masses, might be received in proof of their serving to this transmission; even had we not the more explicit proof of functions impaired or destroyed by injury to the conducting nerves, or to the nervous centres in which they have their origin or termination. Experiments, variously repeated, fully concur with pathological facts in showing how the nervous influence may be thus

---

* Modern science, in its relation to the imponderable elements, has in great degree disengaged itself from those grosser material terms, the use of which was often a serious hindrance to just scientific conclusions. On the other hand, however, much caution is needed that we do not let our reason lose itself in metaphysical abstractions to which no real meaning can be attached. The terms of *force, centres of force,* and *lines of force,* are well justified as the expressions of physical facts. But *force* cannot be understood in the abstract, or apart from *something acted upon;* and we lose all value and sense of the phrase in such manner of its application.

partially or completely arrested.   And the demonstration, so afforded, of an action transmitted through space, and by means of a definite structure, is further enforced by all other phenomena coming under our cognisance.

Admitting, however, this agent of nervous power, the question still presses upon us as to its mode of transit through the nerves; whether by passage of a current, according to the common notion of electrical transmission; or by movements within some part of the nervous structure, having more kindred with those which enter into the undulating theory of light.   This question (closely related to the one we have been considering, but more definite in form,) requires notice here in its bearing upon all that regards the other properties or conditions of nervous agency.   It might seem, for instance, on the latter hypothesis, that we could not rightly speak of the *quantity* of this power, its excess or deficiency, — terms which we shall afterwards find are almost forced upon us to express the notions which the phenomena suggest. Reasoning strictly, however, and with constant reference to the analogy of the other great agents, the inquiry may be prosecuted in similar way, under either of the views just mentioned.   In the science of Electricity, and in those of Light and Heat, the phenomena admit of a double interpretation, beyond what might be deemed possible without knowledge of the facts.   In each of these cases, however, certain of the higher conditions of inquiry are better satisfied on one hypothesis than on the other; and the same thing may eventually happen in our researches regarding the nervous element.   Meanwhile, the expression which best accords with our actual knowledge is that of a

T

power originating within the system, and transmitted *progressively* along the course of the nerves, to fulfil its functions in the several parts of the body to which they conduct ; and through the nerves of sensation and voluntary action, more especially, establishing the relation (as far as we can follow or denote this) between the mind and the material organisation which surrounds it.*

Here, however, we are again called to the question started in the outset, but deferred to this place in the

---

* While speaking on these obscure questions, I cannot forbear adverting to certain results of modern inquiry, closely related to them all, and at the same time ranking among the greatest attainments of the science of our time. I allude here, first, to the recent discovery of molecular changes in the interior of bodies, in effect of the action of heat, electricity, &c., without any alteration of exterior form, density, or chemical composition. The fact that, in some cases, this change and *inter-penetration* of particles is made known to us through optical phenomena (as by alteration in the optical axes of crystals), is in itself a striking evidence of the refinements of modern inquiry, and still more of the establishment of those connexions between the different sciences which have helped to solve so many of the most profound problems in all.

Closely associated in every way with this discovery is another result of still higher interest to physical science ; viz., the extension of the *principle and laws of polarity* to the material actions of all the great elementary forces of nature. Even with our experience of what has already been gained from this source, it would be difficult to divine all that may be attained in the future. The principle is one equally universal and profound, embracing all the forms of matter and action which surround us in the universe ; and associating them, from the greatest to the smallest, under common laws, which are ever tending more and more to the character of mathematical truths.

I advert to these topics, though seemingly separate from our subject, because it is here chiefly that we must look for any relations which may subsist between the powers acting through the nervous system, and the other powers or forces of nature.

argument: — whether we can reason, or attain any sure
result, upon the supposition of a single agent, where the
functions performed differ thus widely in their nature?
We are still unprovided with an absolute answer on this
point. That which is in itself obvious to no sense, and
defined only by certain observed effects, is not easily thus
discriminated; and we must be satisfied with present conclusions of more general kind. The presumption I think
to be in favour of its unity, under such interpretation of
the term as we are reasonably able to give. It will occur
as an obvious argument to this effect, that if we admit
more than one agent in reference to the diversity of offices
fulfilled, we must, by parity of reason, admit several — a
condition very improbable, though we cannot absolutely
disprove it. A second and strong argument is the apparent identity of structure in that portion of the nervous
system, from which we have cause to believe the nervous
power to be evolved. If to these reasons we add the
general uniformity of the minute nervous tissue even of
the sentient and motor nerves, — the connexion of nerves
of different classes with each other and with common
centres, — the apparent provision made by ganglia and
otherwise, for modifying the action in its progress, — and
the equal exhaustion of nervous power by excess of actions
the most diverse in kind, — we may justly infer that it is
an element of single nature with which we are dealing ; —
capable of similar relations of quantity and intensity ; of
like translation to different organs along the course of
nerves; and of suspension by the same causes of injury or
disturbance.

In discussing this question of identity we have to consider, not solely the agent transmitting power, but also the diversity of the organs receiving it. The same influence directed to parts of different composition and structure will produce different results. That which acts in a given manner upon the contractile muscular fibre must be presumed to have other effect upon membranous or glandular organisation. Here again our attention is forcibly drawn to the analogous conditions of electricity; which agent, in its various modes of excitement, conduction, and action on different forms of matter, offers the same class of problems for solution; and, through them, arguments of similar character for the unity of the nervous power. Whether the identity of the two agents can be inferred from any evidence beyond such analogies, is a question we shall speedily have to consider.

Of the several properties or conditions we may assign to the nervous power, that of *Quantity* is, perhaps, the most determinate. The terms of *excess* and *deficiency, exhaustion* and *reparation*, familiar in medical use, seem to be warranted in fact, as well as for the common expression of bodily states or feelings; and scarcely indeed can we explain a single phenomenon of the animal or organic functions without the virtual admission of this idea. Though still unpossessed of any certain proof as to the structure or living actions by which nervous power is generated, yet does this deficiency in no wise alter or affect the inference. It is certain from observation that the production takes place chiefly in the central organs; and, as we have seen, presumably in the cortical or cineritious part of their structure. A constant supply from the generating organs to the conducting nerves is proved to be necessary, to maintain the efficiency of the latter in ministering to all the peculiar actions, single or sympathetic, of animal life. Even as regards the system of nerves of organic life, though apparently endowed with some appropriate nervous power, independent of that of the cerebro-spinal system, yet is this in various ways subordinate to the latter; and requiring a certain amount of constant communication both with it, and with the cerebral hemispheres, to maintain its actions unimpaired. However obscure these relations, they all involve, in one part or other, the notion of quantity; not indeed so definitely as in the case of the voluntary functions; but still admitting no other distinct interpretation of facts.

Of quantity, considered in this general sense, the best exponents are simple excess and deficiency, in as far as they are obvious to us. We have indeed multiplied proofs of the existence of these respective states in all the functions of life. But we are again met here by the difficulty alluded to in the early part of this Chapter, of distinguishing between that supposed sensorial energy, or influence, derived from the higher animal functions and thence pervading the whole system, — and the nervous power or force of which we are now discussing the nature and manner of action. I have already stated our incompetency to deal with all the abstractions of this question. Though the notion of identity cannot easily be maintained, and some authors have separated them even as widely as matter and spirit, yet is it difficult to adapt language to the separate description of their properties and influence. As respects especially the conditions just named, of excess or deficiency, there seems a necessity for applying the same terms to both; nor can we reason upon the phenomena without such admission, even as respects the mental faculties strictly so called.

Confining ourselves, however, to the simplest expression of facts, it is certain that there are constant variations in the amount of that power by which the mind and the animal functions at large are maintained in activity, and associated with the bodily organs and with the world without. These variations occur among different individuals, forming in part what may be considered the temperament of each. But they are still more strikingly manifested in the same individual at different times, and under the different incidents of life. The deficiency of power is what we most familiarly recognise; expressed in ordinary cases by the simple sense of fatigue or exhaustion of those functions, of which the cessation of action is the appropriate repair—in other instances by that more sudden collapse or loss of power, of which every one has occasional experience; sometimes without obvious cause; sometimes, and more remarkably, under the accidents of disorder or disease.

Such deficiency, whatever its degree, may manifestly arise either from a defective production of the power, or from excess in the expenditure of it. The first of these causes, though we have every reason to regard it as largely operative, is more obscurely known to us than the other. While conjecturing with some assurance the structure in which this production occurs, we have no direct evidence as to the manner in which the function is performed, or the modifications it undergoes. Yet from analogy of other organs, we have every right to conclude that quantity forms one of these modifications, and probably a principal one. As the action, under certain conditions, ceases altogether, we must suppose various intermediate states, the effects of which cannot easily be expressed or understood but by this term, or some other equivalent to it. In disease, especially, as might be anticipated, we have frequent presumptive proof of this deficient evolution of nervous power; forming in many cases the most obvious and critical symptom. And the cause of the defect is often more expressly indicated in such cases, by the fact of its occurrence at a time when the expenditure of the power is much below that of the healthy state.*

Still, as I have said, the evidence is more direct of the failure of nervous power from excess in those actions to which it ministers — a physiological fact of great interest in relation to the whole economy of life. For the mental as well as the bodily functions are concerned in this general law of expenditure and reparation; and though the

---

* I find in my notes two or three singular cases, in which (the degree and duration of the symptoms differing in each) there existed what could only be interpreted as a deficiency of nervous power; without any obvious bodily disorder except what this deficiency produced, and unconnected with any aberration of mind; but testified by a general torpor of all the functions of both. In the most remarkable of these cases, (where the symptoms, coming gradually upon a vigorous frame of body, lasted for several months) all the voluntary movements of walking, speaking, eating, &c., were in a sort of abeyance — the mind inert, as if unable to force itself into any effort of thought or feeling — the circulation very feeble — and great torpor of the natural functions. The cessation of this state was as gradual as its commencement, and as little explained by any obvious cause.

system of organic life is much more obscurely dependent upon it, yet even here we find that connexion maintained which seems essential to the unity of the being. Examples might be endlessly multiplied from every organ and action of animal life; expressing by this common effect (as I have before remarked) the probable unity of the agent thus concerned in all. Those connected with sensation and volition are the most important as well as most familiar to us. Every protracted exercise of the senses, especially if too intent in kind, is followed by a feeling of inability and fatigue; — the power gradually ceases which is needed for the distinct perception of objects without. The violent or protracted exercise of the voluntary organs, as in muscular action, has similar and still more obvious effect; — the power is impaired in proportion to the demand upon it. In each case something is consciously felt to be lost, which time and rest are required to regain. Experience tells us, moreover, (and the fact is important), that we cannot, under the fatigue of one sense or function, find fresh and unimpaired force in another. The loss of power, with some certain qualification, is common to all, whatever be the cause producing it; and the manner of reparation is equally so. Relief to the fatigue of one set of muscles may indeed be got by transferring action to another; but this condition is probably connected rather with the proper contractility of the muscular fibre than with the nervous energy bringing it into action.

In speaking of the exhaustion of this power from excess of sensation, I might adduce the effects of simple pain, as an example in point. The fact in question is familiar to every medical man; and especially exemplified in the collapse which frequently ensues upon surgical operations; a due regard to which has of late so beneficially modified the treatment pursued in these cases. The sleep which often instantly supervenes on the cessation of pain (as in the intervals of a protracted labour) affords another testimony to the same effect. In reasoning on these cases, however, we must advert to the fact that the degrees of pain can rarely be estimated by any apparent similarity of lesion or exciting cause. The *sentient state* of the individual is also concerned in the result, — varying much in different persons, and in the same person at different times; though whether this variation depends on the sentient extremities of the nerves, on the ganglia at the root of the sensitive columns, or on the relative amount of the nervous power, can hardly be determined by any evidence we yet possess.*

This part of the subject is one of great interest both to the physician and to the physiologist; and especially since the discovery of those singular properties of Ether, Chloroform, and other anæsthetic agents, which may be said to interpose a barrier for the time between impressions on the sentient nerves, and the perceptions of the sensorium; thus effecting a sort of analysis of one of the greatest functions of the nervous system. Strictly considered, however, these phenomena are not more wonderful in kind than the closely analogous conditions of sleep, of which I have so largely spoken in a former Chapter. All the essential

* Some of the researches by which the discovery of Sir C. Bell has been verified and extended, would seem to show that these ganglia are especially concerned; and a particular observation of Mr. Newport concurs more expressly to the same inference.

incidents of change are the same, and presumably depend on similar physical causes, altering the ordinary transmission of the nervous power.   The state induced by Chloroform is in reality one of the many modifications of this great function of our nature; made more impressive by the manner and suddenness of its occurrence, and by the completeness of that particular effect, which has been happily converted to such large and beneficial use.

Other arguments in addition might be used to sanction the idea of *quantity* in the nervous power, as expressed by its deficiency.   May we not under this view find explanation of the great exhaustion (sometimes involving dangerous results) which follows sudden or excessive growth of the body ; regarding such debility as the effect of disproportion between the size of the frame, and the amount of nervous force ministering to its functions ?*   If there be some ambiguity in this case, for reasons mentioned in the subjoined note, there is less in another instance, which will be familiar to the consciousness of every one.   This is, the sort of measure or estimate we make to ourselves, in any voluntary effort, of the amount of force requisite to fulfil it.   Where the act is one frequently repeated, this can be done with great exactness; but when of unaccustomed kind, there is very often a miscalculation as to the power put forth, and the act fails of being perfectly performed.

---

* In such cases, however, we are bound to advert also to the want of proportionate growth in the muscular structure of the heart, and its consequent inability to carry on an active and healthy circulation, through a vascular system thus unduly extended.   I have seen some very striking examples of this disproportion ; and it is a point in pathology meriting more attention than it has received.

It may further be noticed that when any sudden or violent effort is intended, but desisted from at the instant of execution, there occurs what we may venture to term *a revulsion of unemployed power;* disturbing for a time the whole system by a sort of nervous agitation, greater or less in proportion to the amount of effort which has thus been frustrated of effect. Here again, while admitting a doubtful interpretation, we still recognise the general proof of quantity as an element in nervous power.

Though we cannot except the purely intellectual functions from the influence which thus affects all acts of sensation and volition, yet is the evidence of relation here less definite and certain in application. What we may affirm generally is, that any condition of intent thought or of profound emotion, if long protracted, produces an exhaustion of power, corresponding with that of the bodily organs; and so far allied to it in kind, that the fatigue of the one class of functions prevents more or less for a time the active exercise of the other. Rest from action, and sleep, are the common and sole repair of both. Among all the functions of life, indeed, Sleep is that which best illustrates the facts we have been describing. Its main purpose is obviously that of restoring the nervous power, exhausted by previous bodily or mental effort. The amount required depends on the degree of this exhaustion. The completeness of the restoration afforded is in proportion to the completeness of the sleep. Of the numerous illustrations which occur here, some have been already given in preceding Chapters; but there are many and equally remarkable to which, under the limited plan of my work, I must content myself with simply adverting, as full of curious instruction in this part of physiology.

The same restriction I must follow in considering the effects of *excess* in the amount of nervous power; though this is a point which has not, I think, had due attention given to it, either in the theory or treatment of disease. It is indeed less familiarly recognised than the case of *deficiency;* but yet is clearly attested by various phenomena, and probably by many which are not usually thus interpreted. Admitting the generation of such power by a living action, this deviation from the natural state must be presumed to occur either by excess of production, or by default of expenditure upon the several functions to which it ministers.* Many examples might be cited, common to the consciousness or observation of all, where the augmentation, slight in degree, is testified only by effects perfectly compatible with health — increased sensibility, and greater energy of the active powers both of body and mind, but still under control of the will. These natural effects pass, by a series of gradations, into the more extreme cases which constitute disease; and I cannot doubt that various morbid states, not usually recognised in this light, are really due to excess of that which is the element of nervous power. Among these gradations many cases occur where there seems a necessity for disposing of such excess of nervous energy; — by common exercise of the muscles, where

---

* Though in some of the points here discussed, we come into a sort of proximity to the Brunonian doctrine, yet no argument will be found to warrant the opinions which have borne this name, and which at one time had so much influence in the schools both of Italy and Germany.

it is slight in amount — but in other instances, where the excess is morbid in degree, by violent and spasmodic muscular acts which suddenly expend or give an outlet to the force.   During the vigour of childhood and youth we often have evidence of the former, in an irrepressible desire for action and movement, without other motive than that of satisfying what seems a bodily necessity.*   In a Chapter of my former work (On Morbid Actions of Intermittent kind) I have treated at length of cases of the latter class; adducing instances in Epilepsy, Chorea, and other Spasmodic disorders, where the notions of accumulation, excess, and sudden expenditure are needfully involved; and interesting, moreover, as examples of this power, so affected, passing in great degree out of the control of the will.   This is, under all points of view, an important question in pathology; and the principle, if sanctioned by observation, will explain many things heretofore obscure, in the whole class of spasmodic diseases. We learn, for instance, why there is not only inutility, but even danger, in suddenly and forcibly arresting some spasmodic actions, as those of epilepsy and chorea; and why, in periodical attacks of this kind, there is a ratio often very strikingly maintained between the length of interval and the severity of the succeeding attacks; — each of these

---

* The nervous tricks of children (which, aggravated in degree, become cases of actual Chorea) will often best admit of this explanation; confirmed by the fact that the suppression of one such habit is generally followed by the growth of another.   Little is gained by mere admonition or bodily constraint in these cases.   The progress of age, and direction of the active powers of life to new objects, will do much more to remove the disorder.

cases betokening a cause in which quantity is concerned as an essential element.

Without further repeating those instances, another question occurs here (also alluded to before), whether certain states of mental derangement may not be owing to, or modified by, this excess of nervous power? In Mania, especially, some of the symptoms might well receive this explanation ; such as, the excited sensibility and irrepressible vehemence of action ; the protracted muscular exertions without proportionate fatigue ; and the endurance of long-continued wakefulness without obvious suffering. If we admit this production of excess in any case, there can be no reason to limit it to the condition of a sudden or transient occurrence. The morbid actions implied to account for it, may assume a more chronic form; and continue thus for long periods to disturb the organs and functions submitted to their influence..

From the question of quantity (thus important, as we have seen, to the illustration both of health and disease), we come to certain other more obscure inquiries regarding the nervous power. The question as to *intensity* is the first of these. Whether, in any intelligible sense, we can speak of this as a property distinct from quantity, is very doubtful. The analogy to another imponderable agent, like electricity, must not seduce us too far into inferences, to which language often lends a false appearance of reality. Though we have no just cause to deny the possibility of intensity as a separate attribute, yet neither have we any sufficient reason to affirm it; and the question seems one hardly capable of solution, unless we should hereafter succeed in identifying the elements of nervous force and electricity.

The same obscurity belongs to the notion of *quality*, as applied to the nervous power.   If conceiving of this power as a physical element, derived from or generated by the blood, we must admit the possibility that there may be diversities of property corresponding with changes in the fluid in which it originates.   But the very terms here employed show how vague such conception is ; and we may better serve the interests of science by separating the question from others which are more clearly defined in their objects and methods of pursuit.

To the latter class belongs the question regarding *time*, as a condition in the actions of the nervous power.   In two preceding Chapters I have discussed this in reference to the mental functions ; and recognising in the present case an agency conveyed through nerves, to and from the central organs of the nervous system — capable, moreover, of being arrested, or conducted into different channels, in its course — we must conceive it possible that there may be inequalities in the rate of motion, at different times or in different nerves.   Arduous as this inquiry may appear, the zeal and resources of modern science have applied themselves to its solution.   The recent experiments of M. Helmholtz, of Kœnigsberg, to which reference is made in the subjoined note, have opened the research by very ingenious and refined methods of observation ; and though repetition is needed to confirm the results, we have some cause to consider the principle as actually established.*

---

* These experiments are recorded in a Note transmitted through Baron Humboldt, to the Académie des Sciences, and published in the

Should this eventually prove so, it will be a new and admirable instance of those refinements of research, giving almost a mathematical character to facts which, though obtained by human intellect, far transcend every power of human conception; while by making one great elementary power the index to another, they suggest relations bearing strongly on the unity of all.

In considering these general attributes of the nervous power, a question of much interest still occurs to us; viz., whether this element, so generated within the living body, and distributed to all parts of it in connexion with their several functions, is capable of any kind or degree of diffusion beyond this limit, so as to produce direct influence on other living organisation without? Or, to obviate the ambiguities of language, we may generalise the question, and ask whether any principle of life can, by such mode of communication, be thus directly transferred from one body to another? We must not assert this to be in itself impossible; and one or two high authorities have affirmed its probability. But a fair regard to the proofs alleged will show them to be ambiguous in many

---

" Comptes Rendus," vol. xxx. 1850, entitled " *Sur la vitesse de propagation de l'Agent Nerveux dans les Nerfs Rachidiens*." They appear to have been made with great exactness, by aid of very delicate galvanic apparatus, and with much attention to eliminate all sources of error. As the result of these researches, M. Helmholtz considers the fact to be established, that a *space of time admitting of valuation* is required for the nervous force to pass from the sciatic plexus to the gastro-cnemius muscle in the leg of a frog. Taking the average of his experiments, he found that in a length of nerve of from 50 to 60 millimetres, the time required for transmission (*à parcourir cet espace*) was from 0·0014 to 0·0020 of a second.

very essential points, and admitting of explanation from other and more familiar sources; while there is a strong presumption against the opinion from the absence of all such certain evidence; whereas, if true, proofs to this effect might be looked for, constantly and unequivocally, in every part of life.*

From these topics we readily pass to a question, which has furnished material for discussion to the most eminent physiologists, and is still awaiting the possible solution of future research, viz., the true nature of the agent fulfilling these great functions in the economy of life. Is it one that can be supposed identical with any of those surrounding us in nature, or must we admit at once that it has no type elsewhere in creation? This question is brought more within our scope, by being limited in effect to electrical agency; physiologists having adopted this as rendering the only plausible account of the phenomena. Nor can it excite surprise that they should have been so prone to assume this great element as the moving principle in

---

* The alleged proofs are chiefly furnished by the Mesmerists, to whose views this principle is necessary as a basis; though, as we have elsewhere noticed, they carry the scope of their belief infinitely beyond; making the transmitted energy evolve powers in the recipient which are in no sort possessed by the person communicating it, and which nothing but direct miracle could produce or explain.

Early in the 17th century the sect of Rosicrucians made similar pretensions to the power of curing diseases, &c. by the mysterious action of one human body upon another. In truth, the same or analogous influence has been offered to belief, under one name or other, in every age — differing in the means employed, but singularly alike in the alleged nature of the results, and in the temperament of the persons liable to be thus affected.

the nervous system ; seeing the vastness, or almost universality, of its operation throughout nature ; and the actual
proofs of its intimate and various relations to this part of
the animal economy. Followed through new modes of
development, and tested by more certain and delicate
instruments, it has been found in some cases evolved and
concentrated by vital actions ; — in others, exciting, modifying, or even apparently supplying, the place of these
actions in the body ; — while, regarded in its relation to
heat, to chemical action, and to the whole doctrine of
affinities and polarities, it has the aspect of connecting
together the phenomena of animal and organic life more
completely and naturally than any other principle we can
assume.

It would be impossible for me to pursue into details the
controversy which still exists on this question ; or the
numerous and remarkable experiments which have been
applied to its solution. Collecting generally the results
of these, we must admit that no equivocal proof of identity has yet been attained ; but that the tendency of all
inquiry is towards a closer approximation of the two
elements, and that much cause has been shown, and foundation laid, for further research. Were this to be successful, the result might well rank foremost among the
physical discoveries of our time.

The terms of the question may be briefly stated thus :
Do the various and undoubted effects of electricity in
exciting muscular contraction through the nerves depend
upon the impulse it gives to the motions of the nervous
power ? or are these effects a proof that the agent is really
the same, though generated in different way, and brought
into action by other methods and combinations ?

The main argument against identity is, that electricity, under the form of the voltaic current or otherwise, can continue its excitement to muscular action through a nerve divided, or injured in such manner, that the proper nervous influence is wholly arrested in its course. This argument, strong in the precision of the fact, cannot well be obviated but by assuming a different form of electricity from any yet known, as that generated and acting in the animal frame — an assumption not warranted by other evidence, though rendered plausible by the various modifications of this agency, familiar to us in the electricity of the machine, of the voltaic battery, of the magnet, of thermo-electric combinations, and of electrical fishes. The latter phenomenon, however, which seems on first view a strong evidence of identity, loses its weight as such, by the ascertainment of the peculiar apparatus of nerves and cells existing in these animals; providing for an electrical function wholly distinct from any attribute of the nervous power, and closely resembling those effects of accumulation, tension, and discharge which we obtain by various artificial means.*

* This objection, however, must not be deemed by any means conclusive. Looking to the several forms in which we can excite electricity by the agency of different apparatus, it is very conceivable that its evolution and action as nervous force, may be provided for by other means than those which are required for the larger accumulation or sudden discharge of the power.

We must the rather acquiesce in these subordinate difficulties of proof, seeing that it is still a *vexata quæstio* with philosophers whether electrical currents and polarities can, or cannot, in any case, be excited by simple contact, without the intervention of chemical action — a question fundamental in theory, and, while yet unresolved, giving object and energy to further research.

Though some eminent physiologists have sought to obviate the difficulty, yet is it an argument of weight against the theory in question, that similar muscular contractions are produced by other stimuli, mechanical or chemical in kind, without any certain proof that electricity is evolved or put into action by them. It had always, until lately, been felt as a still stronger negative argument, that by no manner of experiment, however delicate the methods and apparatus employed, could an electric current be detected, as proceeding from muscles in the act of contraction. The researches of Matteucci and Person — valuable in all that concerns the influence of electricity on the nervous and muscular tissues, under every mode of application — fail as to this essential point of evidence; and, if settling the question of identity at all, do so in a negative sense. More recently, however, the experiments of M. Du Bois Reymond, of Berlin, have given a new aspect to this argument. By the use of a most delicate galvanoscope he professes to have obtained distinct deviations of the needle from currents produced by muscular contraction; and these remarkable experiments (repeated before, and reported on by the French Institute) have been certain and constant enough in result, to warrant their being regarded as a distinct physical fact. If admitted as such, they doubtless supply a great void in the evidence; but yet leave the question unresolved as to the identity of the nervous and electric elements. The points still creating doubt I have briefly stated in the subjoined note. They connect themselves mainly with the fact, that in proportion as we make our means of detecting the presence of electrical currents more precise and delicate, in the same proportion do we bring into view the evolution of such currents from causes of physical change, subordinate to, or perhaps wholly distinct from, those which belong to the action of the nervous power.   The importance of this consideration will be readily understood.*

* One main result of the researches of M. Du Bois Reymond may be summarily expressed in the statement, that distinct effects are produced in a galvanometer of extreme delicacy, by the forcible voluntary contraction of the muscles of the fore-arm; a finger on each side being immersed in a vessel of salt water, with which the wires of the galvanometer communicate. Under such arrangement the needle is deflected to one side or the other, according as one or other arm is brought into muscular contraction; the deflection, where the contraction is violent and sudden, occasionally amounting to 50° or 60°, and being *uniform in direction.*

Here, then, is a result so simple and distinct, as seemingly to exclude all other actions than those of the will, the muscular fibre, and the electrical current. Yet, in reasoning upon an agent like electricity,—so universally diffused, and so easily and instantly put into movement by almost every change among material particles,—we are bound to consider whether there be not some action intervening between the muscular contraction, and the electrical current, testified by the needle; — either a chemical change induced in the parts put into contraction — or an alteration of temperature producing a current of thermoelectricity; — or (to go a step further into the obscurity of the subject) whether it may not be, that movements of any kind whatever among the component particles of bodies evolve a certain amount of electricity in an active state; manifest to us when these movements are sufficiently powerful and our instruments delicate enough to give evidence of it.

The experiments and reasoning of Prevost, Dumas, and Edwards, in favour of the electrical theory of nervous power, and the able argument of Müller against it, embody nearly all that could be said on the subject, before the results obtained by Matteucci and Du Bois Reymond had been published. The researches of Dr. W. Philip, in support of the doctrine, were directed to certain of the vital functions; and had there been uniformity of results, or had the same results been obtained by others, his experiment of restoring by a voltaic current

The influence upon the human body of the electrical changes occurring around us in space, have been hitherto very insufficiently studied; seeing the general effects of this great agent upon every form and part of organic life, and its apparently closer relation than that of the other vital stimuli to the functions of the nervous system. On this subject I have treated at length in my former work (Chap. XXVII.), and I do not revert to it here, as the question before us exclusively concerns the supposition of electricity generated or evolved within the body, and not derived from without. Admitting this evolution of animal electricity, independently of all external causes, we might probably best understand it as the effect of those vital actions in which, by chemical change or otherwise, matter is abstracted from, or added to, organs in the discharge of their several functions. But as the doctrine in question presumes these actions themselves to be the effect of electricity in its state of nervous power, we should be admitting the difficult view of operation in a circle; and must rather suppose some more direct mode of generation (of which, it may be, the electrical animals afford the type), and the existence of properties or relations as to intensity, distribution, and manner of influence, of which we have no cognisance in its other forms.

With respect to the Torpedo, Gymnotus, and Silurus electricus (those *Instinctive Electricians*, as they have happily been termed,) it is yet wholly uncertain whether the large nervous ganglia, appropriate to their extraordinary

---

the action of digestion, arrested by section of the par-vagum, might have gone far towards deciding this part of the question.

powers, act directly in producing electricity, or only in giving energy to the extensive organs by which it is accumulated and directed. It is also to be noted that the nerves supplying these organs have very different origin in the three species in question; and, further, that there is no proportion between the intensity of the shock and the size of the nerves in each. These circumstances, indeed, are equivocal in argument; and the latter especially so, from the disparity observed in the different cases between the relative power of giving the shock, of magnetising needles, &c. Under any view, however, of the facts furnished by these singular animals, the question remains yet undecided, whether their electricity is a modification of the nervous power, however produced — or merely evolved by the latter agency, or by other vital actions, and concentrated and directed by the same.*

The doubt then as to the identity of the two great elements of which we are speaking, must still be acquiesced in, while their respective actions remain thus far distinct

---

* The experiments of Dr. Davy on the Torpedo (see his Physiological Researches), and those of Professor Faraday on the Gymnotus (Phil. Trans. 1839), are the most valuable documents we possess on this subject. In the latter part of Professor Faraday's paper are some remarks on the relations of nervous power and electricity, favourable to the view of their virtual identity, and marked by the accustomed sagacity of this philosopher.

I may advert here to those singular instances on record, of persons in whom, at intervals, there occurs such large development of electricity as to show itself in sparks through the skin. Such cases, however, (allowing their authenticity,) do not prove more than the strongly opposed tension of the electricity on the surface of the body to that of objects around; and the rarity of their occurrence further deprives them of any weight in the argument.

to our actual knowledge. If hereafter the affirmative should be proved, it will probably be in the same sense, and as part of the same train of discovery, by which all these great elementary agents of the material world are gradually converging towards a common principle, the highest and ultimate object of human science. Meanwhile it may be affirmed that if any one of the powers of inanimate nature, as we now define them, be concerned in the functions of the nervous system, electricity is indisputably that which best fulfils the conditions required. And while admitting all the difficulties of the question, a fair regard to the progress and actual state of physical science would render it even more bold to affirm these difficulties to be insuperable, than to assert that they will eventually be solved.

Though the preceding review of the course and state of inquiry into the nervous system has embraced a vast variety of topics, there are yet others, which have only partially been noticed, though inseparable from the subject, and of the highest interest in physiology. Such are, especially, the relation of the power acting through this system to the powers of the proper organic life — the most wonderful, perhaps, of all the known links in creation; connecting together, into common functions and effects, principles wholly distinct to our present comprehension. The vital properties of the blood, and those inherent in the muscular fibre (the just definition of which we owe to two physiologists of equal fame) form the main foundation of organic existence as distinguished from inorganic matter; and the modes in which these properties are severally brought into operation by the powers acting through the nervous system, stand foremost among the great problems of physiological science.   Every influence of this system on the matter composing the animal frame must, as far as we can understand, be applied through, or upon, these two media.   And to the same relations we have reason to look for what concerns the phenomena of generation and reproduction; always admitting that we reach but the threshold of this mystery; and that the manner of action of organisation, in giving similar vital properties to inorganic matter, must presumably be for ever unknown.

I have already alluded to the intimate connexion of the nervous and vascular systems; and particularly to that close union in the extreme branches of each, through which it is probable that their most important functions are performed.   A few words still remain to be said respecting the connexion of the nerves with muscular action — a fruitful subject of research, with greater facilities for observation than in the case of the blood, and involving, among other topics, one of singular interest in the economy of life; viz., the relation of the nervous power to the proper contractility of the muscular fibre.   This inquiry (founded on the distinction which Haller not too strongly designates as a *lex æterna*), includes many subordinate questions, requiring more examination than they have yet obtained.   Such questions principally regard the varying proportion which the nervous and muscular powers bear to each other in the numerous phenomena of action, exhaustion, intermission, and reparation.   We have already found reason for estimating the nervous power under the condition of quantity; and the muscular contractility also is of variable amount, depending not alone on its expenditure in action, but also on many other natural or morbid conditions of the body. The two powers are independent and dissimilar; have their origin in different sources; and presumably exist at the same time in very different proportions and capacity for action. The cases and combinations arising out of this relation (multiplied further by the distinction of voluntary and involuntary motions) are doubtless concerned in producing many of those anomalous results which occur to our notice both in health and disease. A more explicit regard to them under this view might probably solve various difficulties which still embarrass the subject.

There are yet other points connected with the physiology of the nervous system, to which, before closing this Chapter, I must briefly advert. One is, the question as to the influence of the brain and nerves in the production of animal heat — an inquiry suggested forty years ago by some remarkable experiments of Sir B. Brodie, and since pursued by other physiologists. The chemical theory on this subject has been more currently adopted, especially since the support given to it by the researches and writings of Liebig; but there is still evidence enough to justify the belief that the nervous system is in some manner concerned in this important function.

Another subject of modern research has been the action of different poisons upon the brain and nerves; an inquiry which abounds in singular and inexplicable results. Here, again, we are indebted to some early experiments of Sir B. Brodie, which have been extended and varied by later physiologists; indicating especially the distinction between those poisons which produce death indirectly through other parts, and those which are fatal by direct and instant action on the nervous system.   The experiments of MM. Bernard and Pelouze on the Curare poison are the most recent and remarkable we possess on this subject.   Acting through the blood, but so instantaneously as to preclude all theory of fermentation or change in that fluid (of which the fertile genius of Liebig has made such large use in other cases), this poison at once annihilates the nervous power.   In animals killed suddenly by other means, the nerves retain their irritability for longer or shorter time; — where death is produced by this substance, they are wholly unaffected by the strongest stimuli.   I select this as one of the most striking examples of the influence of certain organic agents on that portion of animal life, which gives power and vitality to the rest; — an influence the more wonderful from the minute quantity of the agent; and from a chemical composition so closely akin to that of substances wholly innocuous, that the abstraction or addition of a single component atom often makes the sole difference between an aliment and a poison.   Organic Chemistry has disclosed these marvellous changes in the intimate structure of bodies, though it utterly fails in explaining to us how they can thus instantly affect the principle of life.

In closing this Chapter I must again remark that the topic is that to which all separate researches in physiology converge ; blending themselves in this common centre — on the one hand, with the higher doctrines of life, reproduction, and mental existence — on the other, with those great general powers or laws of inanimate nature which are ever in action within and around us.   Physiological

science, on the matter in question, seems at this moment
to be on the verge of some greater discovery; resembling
in this respect the actual state of other physical sciences
— those of light, heat, electricity, chemical forces, and
perchance gravitation — which the course of modern inquiry is ever tending to reduce to certain common laws.
It is a question of deep interest, already referred to, whether the relation here is not closer than that of mere
analogy ; and whether future research may not associate
some of the functions of the nervous system with the more
general elements of force and action in the physical world.
Vital laws, and what we term physical laws, stand precisely in the same relation to our knowledge.   They are
continually approximating as this knowledge advances ;
and may not impossibly in the end be submitted, even in
human comprehension, to some common principle, embracing the whole series of phenomena, however remote
and dissimilar they now appear.*

   All science tends to prove the unity of creation, through
the evidence it affords of mutual and universal relation of
parts.   The expression of an eminent philosopher, —
" L'univers, pour qui sauroit l'embrasser d'un seul point

---

   * Since 1839, when this passage was written, much has been done
to confirm these anticipations, and to extend inquiry into that region
of general laws, towards which so many separate paths now converge.
The suggestions derived from every part of physical science, and
especially from the admirable researches of Faraday, on the mutual connexion of the elementary forces, have been methodised and enlarged
by Professor Grove, in a remarkable treatise on " the Correlation of
Physical Forces ;" while Dr. Carpenter has given further extension
to the same views, by a paper on " the Mutual Relations of the Vital
and Physical Forces," published in the " Phil. Trans. for 1850."

de vue, ne seroit qu'un fait unique et une grande vérité," though in one sense it may seem a vague imagination, yet, in a larger scope of view, involves the great result and term of all philosophy.   The " single fact " and " great truth," is that of one Almighty Cause ; — a conclusion to which we are irresistibly carried forwards from every side; surmounting in this inference those intermediate gradations of existence and power, which are too dimly seen to be rightly apprehended by the faculties of man in his present state of being.

THE END.

LONDON:
SPOTTISWOODES and SHAW,
New-street-Square.